Conception to Confinement

Facts an Antenatal Mother should Know

DR. SEETESH GHOSE & DR. NIKITA

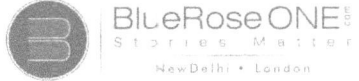

BLUEROSE PUBLISHERS
India | U.K.

Copyright © Dr Seetesh Ghose & Dr Nikita 2023

All rights reserved by author. No part of this publication may be reproduced, stored in a retrieval system or transmitted in any form or by any means, electronic, mechanical, photocopying, recording or otherwise, without the prior permission of the author. Although every precaution has been taken to verify the accuracy of the information contained herein, the publisher assume no responsibility for any errors or omissions. No liability is assumed for damages that may result from the use of information contained within.

BlueRose Publishers takes no responsibility for any damages, losses, or liabilities that may arise from the use or misuse of the information, products, or services provided in this publication.

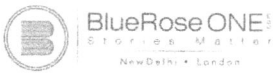

For permissions requests or inquiries regarding this publication, please contact:

BLUEROSE PUBLISHERS
www.BlueRoseONE.com
info@bluerosepublishers.com
+91 8882 898 898
+4407342408967

ISBN: 978-93-5819-718-1

Cover design: Tahira
Typesetting: Tanya Raj Upadhyay

First Edition: November 2023

INTRODUCTION TO THE BOOK

Pregnancy is a physiological process that every woman wishes to undergo. Although 80% of these women will have normal course of pregnancy. But, unless taken care of during antenatal period, these women end up in various pregnancy related complications. To avoid such unwarranted complications all women must have basic knowledge about the conception, progresses of pregnancy and confinement. Although many information is available in this regard, it is an attempt to provide those facts in a comprehensive manner in simple language to the readers. It also gives the important practical tips related to conception, overall antenatal, intra-natal and post-natal care along with contraception or family planning measure.

Hope this book will help every woman, who is contemplating pregnancy or already pregnant, to attain not only a successful pregnancy but also a complete womanhood.

Wish every woman a happy motherhood!!

ABOUT AUTHORS

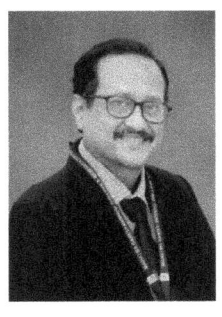

Dr. Seetesh Ghose, MD, Obstetrics and Gynecology, is presently working as Dean and Professor, in the department of Obstetrics and Gynecology at MGMCRI, Sri Balaji Vidyapeeth, Puducherry. He has 26 years of experience and contributed immensely to the academics, patient care and research. His area of interest is high-risk pregnancy, minimal access and reconstructive surgery.

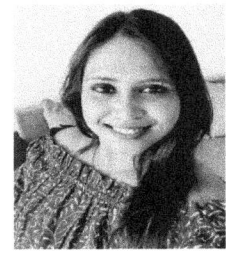

Dr. Nikita, MS, Obstetrics and Gynecology, presently working as an Assistant Professor in the department of Obstetrics and Gynecology in SMMCH, Chennai. She is a multi-talented, dedicated budding O&G consultant. Her area of interest is high risk pregnancy and minimal access surgery. She wishes to work for wellbeing of the women hood.

We thank Dr. Vignesh and Dr. Srisandarsh Uppu for helping us in adding pictures in our book.

TABLE OF CONTENTS

Introduction 1

Process Of Conception or Getting Pregnant 6

Preparation For Pregnancy 12

Development of your baby 18

Antenatal care 22

Investigations in pregnancy..44

Labour, Delivery and Post Delivery Care...................50

Newborn Care..64

Lactation..70

Contraception after delivery..82

common Problems in Pregnancy..................................86

Common Medical Problem during Pregnancy 96

Commonly Asked Question in Pregnancy 104

Myths and Facts Related to Pregnancy....................122

Role of husband in pregnancy care...........................134

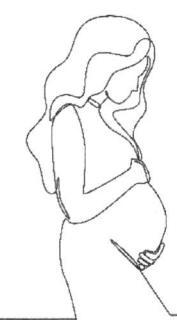

INTRODUCTION

Pregnancy is one of the best things which can happen to a woman. Giving birth to a new life is not an easy task. After seeing those two lines on the urine pregnancy test, you confirm your pregnancy and that feeling is the best feeling a woman can have. There are lots of changes in the body which happen rapidly during pregnancy which makes a woman a little worried. And in today's world where people's attitude is changing towards life in terms of food habits, lifestyle etc. And also, people are getting married late due to their careers. Now there is a trend of "delayed motherhood". However, pregnancy beyond 35 years of age is challenging. Getting pregnant for everyone is not easy now-a-days. Women face many challenges to become pregnant and deliver a healthy baby like they undergo many miscarriages and suffer from many medical diseases during pregnancy like hypertension, diabetes and thyroid etc. However, right from the beginning if you start taking care of your health, take a balanced diet and do exercise regularly. If you take care of your body and mind properly then you can deliver a healthy baby. *Let's get started.*

"A baby is something you carry inside you for nine months, in your arms for three years, and in your heart until the day you die."

— Mary Mason

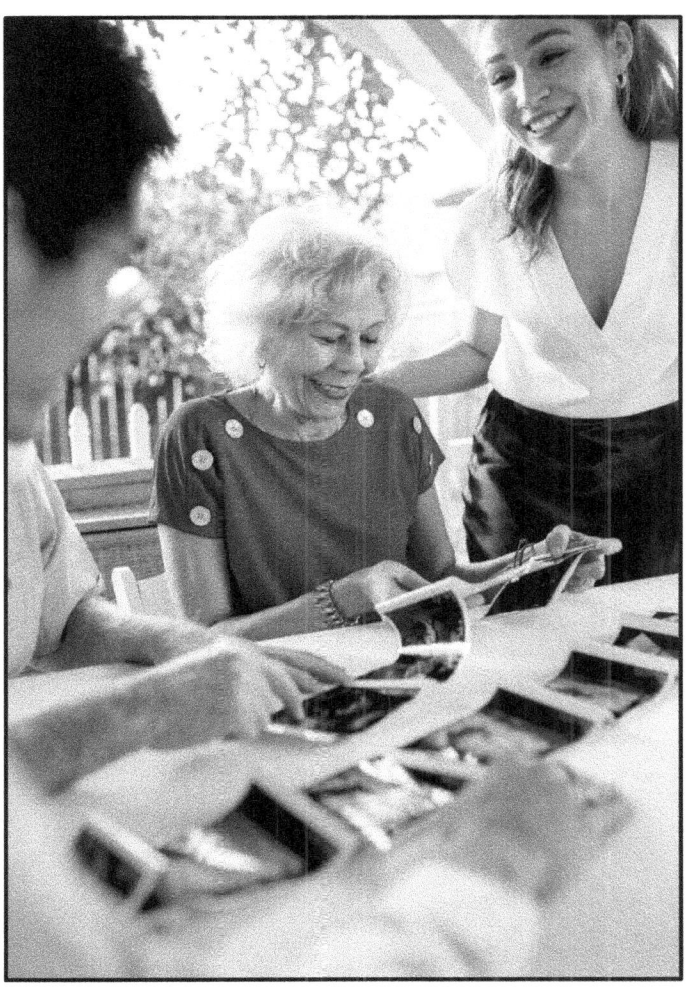

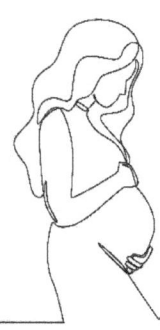

PROCESS OF CONCEPTION OR GETTING PREGNANT

Now let's know step by step biological process of conception or getting pregnant

Conception is the process by which a new human life begins, and it involves several sequential steps. Here is the sequence of conception:

- **Ovulation (Day-1)**: The process begins with ovulation, which is the release of a mature egg (ovum) from one of the ovaries. Ovulation typically occurs around the middle of the menstrual cycle i.e., 14th day of onset your period, provided your menstrual cycle happen regularly every month. Under normal circumstances this mature egg is picked up by fallopian tube.
- **Fertilization (Day 1-6 after ovulation)**: If sperms are present in the female reproductive tract at the time of ovulation, one sperm cell ascents and penetrate and fuses with the egg. This event is known as fertilization. It typically occurs in the fallopian tube.

- **Formation of zygote (Day 2-3 after fertilization):** When a sperm successfully fertilizes the egg, it forms a single-cell structure known as zygote. This zygote now contains the unique combination of genetic material from both the mother and the father.
- **Formation of blastocyst (Day 6-7 after fertilization):** The zygote undergoes rapid cell division, becoming a multicellular structure known as a blastocyst. During this process, the blastocyst continues to travel down the fallopian tube toward the uterus.
- **Implantation (Day 7-10 after fertilization):** The blastocyst eventually reaches the uterus and must implant itself into the uterine lining (endometrium) for further development. Successful implantation involves the attachment of the blastocyst to the uterine wall.
- **Development of the Embryo (2-3 weeks after fertilization):** After implantation, the blastocyst begins to differentiate and develop into an embryo. The embryo goes through various stages of development, eventually forming the three germ layers that give rise to different tissues and organs.
- **Development of the fetus (4-12 weeks after fertilization):** Following implantation these cells grow and differentiate into placenta and fetus. The placenta is an essential organ that allows the exchange of nutrients, oxygen, and waste products between the mother and the developing fetus. It

provides support and nourishment to the growing embryo/fetus.
- **Further development:** Over the course of approximately nine months, the developing embryo/fetus undergoes extensive growth and development, with the various organ systems forming and functioning.
- **Birth:** The final event of the conception happens as birth of a baby. The baby is typically delivered through the mother's birth canal (vaginal birth) or through abdomen by a surgical procedure i.e., cesarean section (C-section).

It's important to note that not every fertilized egg successfully results in a pregnancy or live birth. Many factors can affect the progression and outcome of conception, and there may be instances of early pregnancy loss (miscarriage) or unsuccessful implantation.

Some facts about conception

- For fertilization to occur, sperm should enter the vagina <48 hours prior to ovulation.
- On an average, in one ejaculation men release 2-5 mL of semen. 1mL of semen contains 60-100 million of sperm which means in one ejaculation 200-500 million of sperm is being ejaculated. Of which thousand sperm reach enter into fallopian tube for fertilization of which only one sperm fertilizes the mature ova.

- Window period for fertilization (fertile period)- 48 hours before ovulation to 24 hours after ovulation.
- The lifespan of a female egg is 24 hours whereas sperm's lifespan is 72 hours.
- If you want to get pregnant or you are facing difficulty in getting pregnant then you should plan your intercourse during your fertile period.

Pregnancy symptoms- Symptoms of pregnancy is seen as early as 7-8 days of fertilization. We will discuss in detail about it in later chapters.

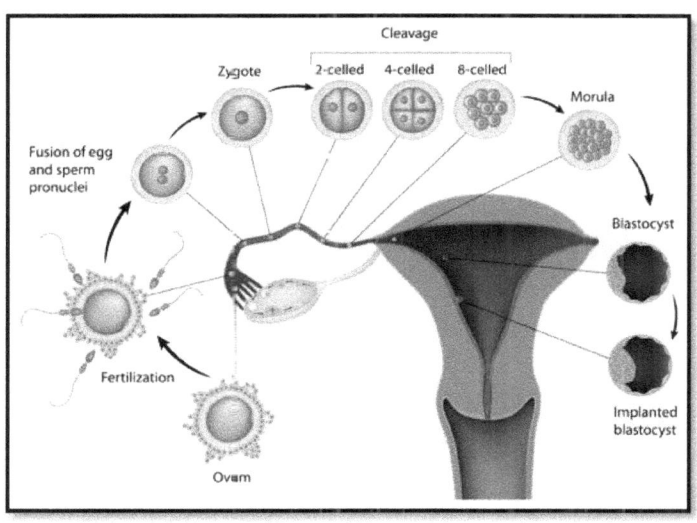

Source: Getting Pregnant: Anatomy & Basic Conception: Tennessee Reproductive Medicine

https://trmbaby.com/library/getting-pregnant/

"Life is a flame that is always burning itself out, but it catches fire again every time a child is born."

— George Bernard Shaw

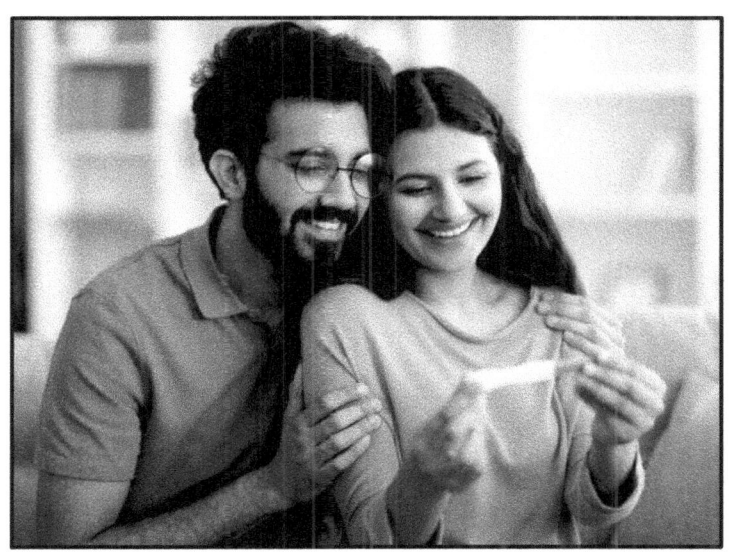

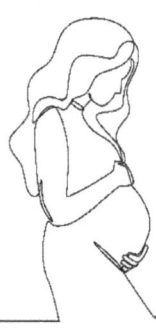

PREPARATION FOR PREGNANCY

(Tips to get pregnant easily)

Always it is better to plan your pregnancy and for that you must track your ovulation. Because, as mentioned in the previous chapter intercourse around ovulation increase your chance of getting pregnant. I have also mentioned, ovulation takes place on 14th day in case of regular cycle (28days) and 14 days prior to next period date in case of longer cycle (>35days). Here are some tips how track ovulation.

Signs of ovulation, that help you to track your time of ovulation.

- **Basal body temperature (BBT):** It's a resting body temperature which rises after ovulation due to release of progesterone hormone. Select a BBT thermometer with two decimal place to provide accurate readings. Measure your BBT at the same time every morning even on weekend and during your menstrual period. The best time to take BBT is upon waking, before getting out of bed and before engaging in any physical activity or even speaking.

Try to minimize any factors that might affect your BBT which include lack of sleep, alcohol consumption (if any), illness, stress or any other condition that can disrupt your sleep pattern. Ovulation typically increase BBT around 0.5-1º F (0.3 to 0.6º C) Your BBT increases 0.5-1 F after ovulation. The limitation of this method is it may not pinpoint the exact day of ovulation with absolute certainty. It is more effective when combined with other methods of tracking ovulation such as cervical mucus or ovulation predictor kit.

- **Cervical Mucus Method:** To do this, look at and/or touch your vaginal discharge to determine its consistency and color. If it is very watery resembles raw egg whites and stretchy i.e., you can stretch it up to 10 cm, then you are likely to ovulate soon. This is due to high level of estrogen during ovulation.
- **Mid-cycle pain:** You may feel lower abdominal pain in the middle of your menstrual cycle (also known as mittelschmerz means middle pain in German). The pain is sharp and sudden, on one side, dull and achy, similar to menstrual cramps. accompanied by slight vaginal bleeding or discharge and rarely, severe. This is due to rupture of follicle and release of ovum.
- Sexual desire increases during ovulation due to increase in level of estrogen and testosterone hormones.

- You may feel breast tenderness, bloating, nausea, headache and mood swing.
- **Ovulation predictor kit**: You can track your ovulation just like urine pregnancy test. Use this kit few days before you think you will ovulate. This kit detects rise in luteinizing hormone (LH) in urine which occurs 24-36 hours prior to ovulation. If this test comes positive you can have intercourse in those 2-3 days.
- **Follicular monitoring ultrasound**: You can meet your doctor for this test. In this test your doctor will assess the growth of your follicles and signs of ovulation in the ovary.

Fertile window- Chances of conception is high five days before ovulation and two days after ovulation as earlier mentioned the life span of ovum is approx. 48hrs and sperm's life span is 72hrs. From day 10th to day 16th, in these seven days you are most likely to conceive. So, you can have intercourse daily or on alternate days during this fertile window.

- **Diet:** Diet plays a main role in conception. Make sure you eat healthy and balanced diet. Eat lots of fruits and vegetables if you are trying to conceive because fruits and vegetables are rich in anti-oxidants which help in fighting harmful free-radicals which damages egg and sperm quality. So, make sure you add seasonal fruits and vegetables in your diet on daily basis. Use wholegrain cereals and eat lots of fiber rich food. Include omega-3 rich food like flaxseeds, walnuts which has positive effect on ovulation and help in production of progesterone hormone. Encourage your husband to take Vitamin E & C rich food like citrus fruits and sunflower seeds which increases sperm count and motility. You should also include iron rich diet like spinach, beans etc. in your diet. Avoid trans-unsaturated fat, instead you can use monounsaturated fat like olive oil. Avoid red meat, sugar, refined carbohydrates, fast food etc.

- **Exercise**: Exercise increases the chance of getting pregnant. If you have lots of body fat then it will produce lots of estrogen which will affect your ovulation. You can go for walking, yoga and keep yourself active. However, avoid strenuous exercise because it will affect your ovulation.
- **Folic acid**: Three months prior to conception you should start taking folic acid. It has tremendous benefits. It improves the embryo quality. It decreases the risk of birth defect in babies like neural tube defects. It prevents organogenesis related miscarriages.
- **Smoking and alcohol**: Quit smoking and alcohol consumption, it affects your ovulation and can affect your egg quality as well.
- **Caffeine**: Make sure you don't take caffeine more than 200 mg per day which is approx. two cups of coffee a day.
- **Stress**: Stress can affect your ovulation so try to keep yourself stress free. Take proper sleep as well.

- **Pre-conceptional counselling / pre-pregnancy checkup:** Visit your doctor for pre-conceptional counselling to have detailed discussion about your overall health and for risk assessment. Your doctor will suggest you if any lifestyle modification needed. Don't forget to tell your doctor about your pre-existing health condition and medication if any, which might affect your pregnancy. Inform your doctor if there is any genetic disease in your family so according to that your doctor will decide whether genetic screening is needed or not.

"Carrying a baby is the most rewarding experience a woman can enjoy."

-Jayne Mansfield

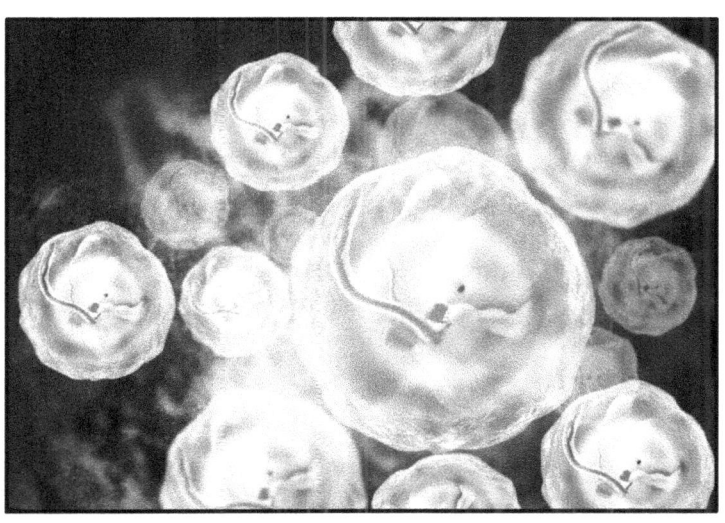

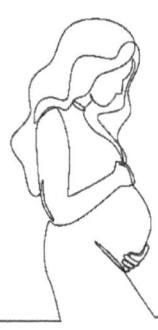

DEVELOPMENT OF YOUR BABY

Let's talk how babies grow inside the womb....

- Before eight weeks, developing baby is called an embryo but from eight weeks it is called fetus.
- Embryo is first detectable by USG when it is around 1-2 mm long and increases in length by 1 mm/day.
- Heartbeat of a baby is seen as early as 37 days of conception when embryo size is 2 mm or more.
- Implantation takes place at three weeks or after 21 days of your periods.
- Between 4-5 weeks embryo settles down in uterus and its size is 5 mm.
- Between 6-7 weeks size from head to bottom is 8-10 mm and heartbeat is visible on ultrasound.
- Between 7-8 weeks, fetus size is 11-16 mm.
- Between 8-9 weeks, fetus size is 17-23 mm and limb buds also appear. Head can be seen separately from the body. The major internal organs i.e., heart, brain, kidneys, gut, liver also develop.
- Between 9-10 weeks fetus size is 23-32 mm. Fetal movements also can be seen.

- After 12 weeks fetus is formed completely. At 14 weeks baby is 85 mm and it's all organ is fully developed.
- Between 15-22 weeks face is more defined, eyebrows, eyelashes and hair start to grow. Your baby is covered with "lanugo", it is soft hair in which baby is covered to maintain its body temperature. It disappears after birth. If it's your first baby, you start feeling the baby's movement between 16-22 weeks. But if this is your second baby then you feel fetal movement little earlier between 16-18 weeks. At this stage fetus size is 27cm.

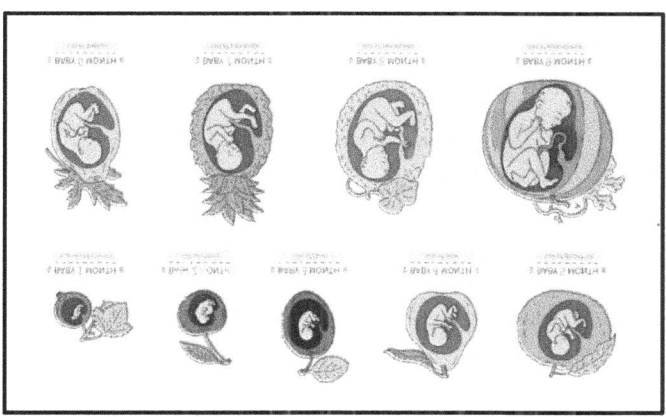

- Between 23-30 weeks fetus responds to sound and touch. Baby moves and kicks when they hear music. They start swallowing and urinating. At 26 weeks your baby opens its eyelids for the first time. Your baby starts getting hiccups. At 30 weeks, your baby is around 33cm.

- At around 32 weeks baby starts descending downwards. If your baby's position is breech (legs downwards) or transverse then at 36 weeks your doctor will repeat scan to look for its head and decide the mode delivery accordingly.

"Giving birth should be your greatest achievement not your greatest fear."

—*Jane Weideman*

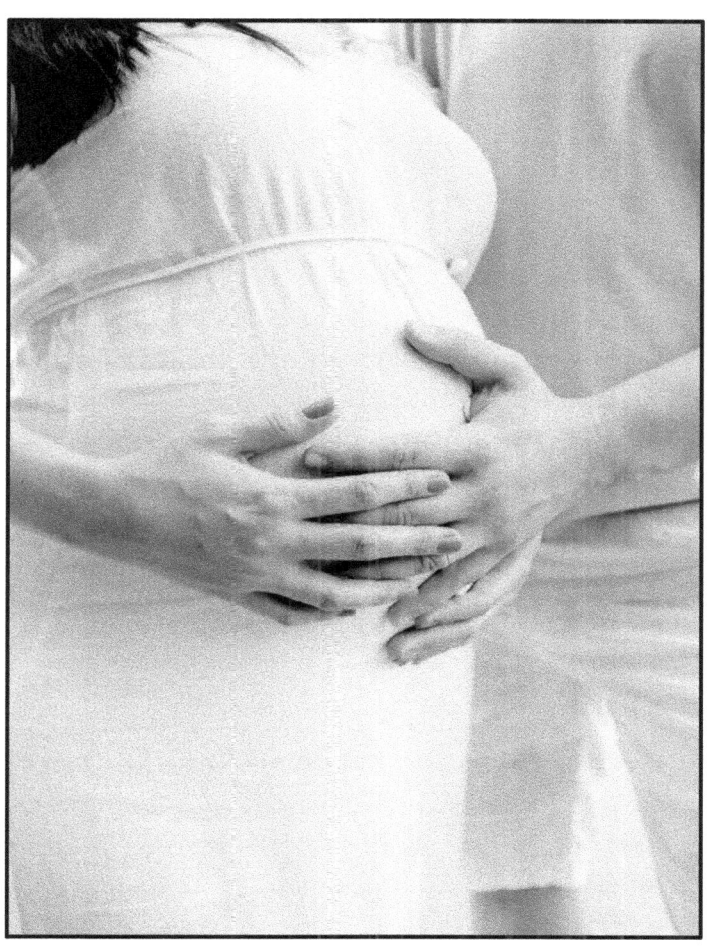

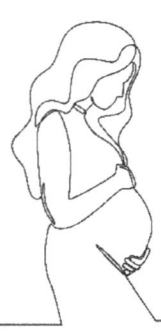

ANTENATAL CARE

The period between conception to till birth of the baby is known as antenatal period. For your successful pregnancy outcome i.e., having a healthy baby at the end of labour process without affecting your health, antenatal care plays an important role. Considering the different physiological changes, requirement of the body and baby's growth whole antenatal period is divided into first, second and third trimester. Each trimester is unique from other in the form of pregnancy presentation, necessary investigation and management wise.

First Trimester

- Pregnancy is so eventful process that the changes are visible in weeks. So, the first trimester indicates the first three months (1-12 weeks) of your pregnancy.
- Your body undergoes lots of changes due to initiation of pregnancy related hormonal changes. It is also crucial period for the structural formation of fetus. Up to 10 weeks this formation of your baby

happens following which growth continues. You should take care of your health properly.

- In first trimester, common complaint is nausea and vomiting which is commonly known as morning sickness in medical term. They generally occur after first or second missed periods and subsides by end of first trimester. 50 % women get both nausea and vomiting, 25% get only nausea and 25% don't have any of these.

Tips to manage nausea & vomiting in first trimester

- **Diet:** Food which triggers the symptoms should be avoided, oily and spicy foods should be avoided. Take frequent small meals. You can take biscuits, dry toast, protein rich diet. You can take ginger whenever you feel nauseating.
- **Medications:** Take Vitamin B1 and B6 supplements.
- If this nausea and vomiting interferes with your daily activities, you should consult your doctor.

Booking

- Don't forget to register yourself to some hospital, it is very important. In first trimester you should visit your doctor at least once.

Investigations in first trimester

- **Blood tests**: Complete blood count, blood glucose test, urine routine, serology (VDRL, HIV, HbS Ag),

blood grouping and typing, thyroid function test. These are basic tests to know your health status.
- **Ultrasonography**: This test is very important and gives lot of information about the baby.
    o You should go for scans in first trimester from 6weeks to 12 weeks. Baby's heartbeat can be seen from 6 weeks. In first trimester scan, doctor will see whether your baby is intrauterine or outside the uterus, whether there is one or two or three fetuses. First scan is known as dating scan or viability scan which can be done abdominally or vaginally. You should not miss this scan. If your menstrual dates are wrong then, with this scan doctor can check your correct expected delivery date also.
    o Second scan is NT scan (Nuchal translucency scan) done between 11+6 to 14 weeks. In this scan doctor sees thickness of the fluid behind the neck of the fetus to rule out any genetic disorder like Down's syndrome and also the anatomy of the baby means how your baby's body parts are growing. This scan is done along with blood test known as dual marker in which two tests are included PAPPA and Beta hCG. This dual marker should be done within 24 hours of NT scan.
- **Medication:** You must take certain supplements as prescribed by your doctor.
    o **Folic acid:** Once you know you are pregnant, you should start taking folic acid 5 mg once in

a day. In fact, you should start taking three months prior to your conception. You should not delay in taking folic acid because it helps in development of nervous system, heart, circulatory system and neural tube of the baby. It prevents defects of brain and spine of baby, also reduces the risk of organogenesis related miscarriages.

- **Dental appointments:** Do not forget to visit your dentist because dental health is as important as physical health. Poor oral health can cause pre-term labour and low birth weight babies etc.

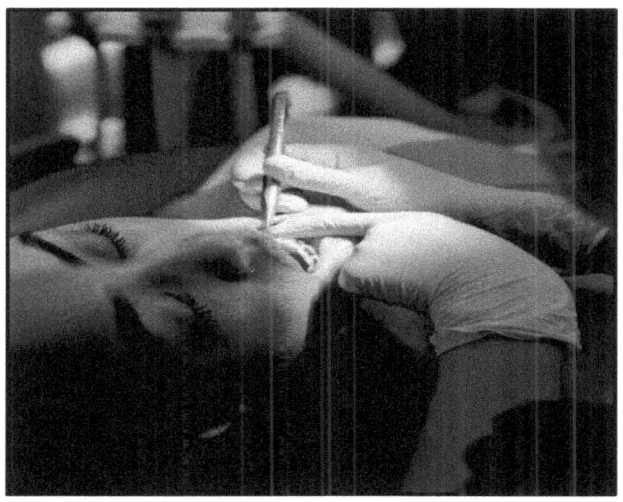

Second Trimester: This is second three month of the pregnancy i.e., 13 to 28weeks.

- o You will start feeling better now. Your nausea and vomiting will reduce.

- You will notice some physical changes in the form of increase in breast size. So, ensure you are wearing right size of bra.
- Your abdomen will increase in size. You need loose clothes.
- You can start feeling your baby's movement. Women pregnant for the first time can perceive fetal movements by 20 weeks and women pregnant for 2nd or 3rd time can perceive fetal movement by 16 weeks.
- You can hear your baby's heartbeat on doppler by 16-20 weeks.
- **Investigations**: In second trimester few important investigations are there. You need to get them done without missing.
  - **Blood**: OGTT at 26-28 weeks if your glucose test were normal in first trimester.
  - **Ultrasonography**: Anomaly scan between 18-22 weeks. In this scan doctor will see how is your baby is growing, how is your baby's organ developing and whether there is any anomaly, resistance in your uterine arteries blood flow and cervical length. This scan is very important, don't miss it.
  - **Fetal ECHO**- If you are diabetic or there is any abnormality in fetal's heart in anomaly scan then you should go for ECHO test to see your baby's heart in detail.
  - If you miss dual marker then you can do quadruple marker test done between 16- 20

weeks. In this test four blood tests are included alpha-fetoprotein (AFP), Beta hCG, unconjugated estriol (uE3) and Inhibin A. This test is also done to rule out genetic disorders like down syndromes.

In second trimester, you must visit your doctor at least once and as and when required by you or as advised by your doctor.

- **Medications:** You must take certain supplements as prescribed by your doctor.
  - Start on iron and calcium tablets from after 12 weeks.
  - Take two doses of TT or Td injection. First dose between 16-24 weeks and after one month take 2nd dose. Some doctors give TT/Td at first visit also.
  - Alternatively, you can take one dose of TT injection and one dose of Tdap (Tetanus, Diphtheria and Pertussis)
  - If you have taken these injections in your previous pregnancy correctly, and the gap between pregnancy is less than 3 years you can take only one booster dose.
  - If you have taken these injections in your previous pregnancy correctly, and gap between pregnancy is more than 3 years you must take two doses of TT or Td injection or one dose of TT injection and one dose of Tdap.

Summary of the TT injection

Previous pregnancy	GAP	Current pregnancy
2 doses of TT	≤3 years	1 dose of TT
2 doses of TT	>3 years	2 doses of TT
No TT doses	Any duration	2 doses of TT

Third trimester

This is the final lap of your happy journey and but very crucial. This is from 29 to 40 weeks. You need to take extra care of yourself.

- **Investigations**: Certain investigations need to be repeated.
  o Ultrasound need to be repeated to assess the growth of the baby between 28-32 weeks This test is done with or without doppler in which blood supply to your baby is seen. At 38 weeks once again growth scan is done to see the position of the baby, liquor and baby's weight.
  o Repeat hemoglobin level and serology at 38 weeks.
- **Fetal monitoring:** Your doctor may use cardiotochogrphy machine to monitor your baby's heart rate which is known as non-stress test (NST).
- **Medications and Vaccines**
  o Continue to take your medicines regularly.
  o Take vaccine Tdap which gives protection against tetanus toxoid, diphtheria and pertussis. It should be taken between 27-36 weeks.

- If your blood group is negative then your doctor will give Anti-D injections between 28-32 weeks. Some doctors give two doses first at 28 weeks and second at 34 weeks.

Now you should start preparing for *'The Day'* (delivery). Get your bag ready which should contain the followings:

- Some 3-4 loose dresses with front opening dresses.
- Tight breast supportive bras at least 3-4 sets.
- Maternal large pads at least one full packet.
- Dresses for baby 3-4 sets.
- Brush, toothbrush, comb, toothpaste, towels.
- Dresses, nappies along with socks and mittens for the baby to keep it warm.
- Books, magazines, laptop or headphones to hear music if you are a music lover.
- Blanket to wrap your baby.
- Any other things that you feel appropriate for you.

- **Diet**: Healthy diet is very important if you are pregnant because your baby needs nutrition to grow. There is no special diet for pregnancy, you just need to eat wholesome and healthy balanced diet because whatever you eat, will pass on to your baby.

Your diet should include fruits, vegetables, rice, bread, milk and if you are non-vegetarian then you can include meat, fish and eggs as well.

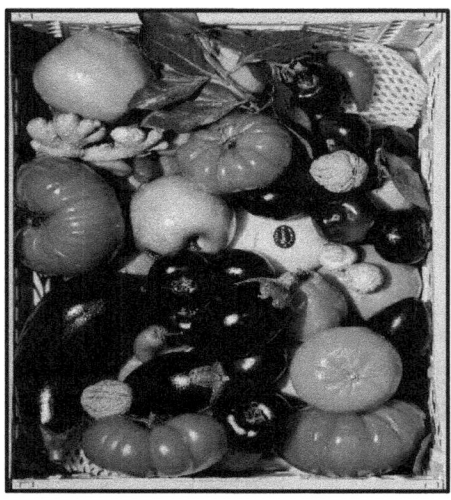

- **Anti-oxidants-** Fruits are rich in anti-oxidant which prevent tissue damage. Fruits are rich in fibers which help in digestion and prevent constipation. In pregnancy, progesterone hormones are in excess which causes constipation so make sure you consume seasonal fruits to avoid constipation. Don't forget to wash them properly before eating.
- **Folic acid -** Source: Green leafy vegetables, broccoli, fruits like oranges, avocado, banana, jaggary, bread and whole grain cereals.

  Benefits:

  o Help in development of nervous system and neural tube.

- Helps in the formation of heart and circulatory system.
- Prevents birth defects like spina bifida and pre-term labour
- Lowers the risk the organogenesis related miscarriages.

- **Iron**

  Source: Wood apple, green leafy vegetables like spinach, beans, lentils, jaggery, drumstick leaves and vegetable, dry fruits, lean meat, chicken, salmon fish.

  Benefits:
  - Iron is an important mineral produced by the body. In pregnancy you need twice as normal 27-30mg/day and if you are anemic then you should take 120mg/day to make more blood to supply oxygen to your baby.
  - It helps in the growth of fetus and placenta.

- **Calcium**

  Source: Dairy products, green vegetables, seafood, peas and beans, fox nut, fish, broccoli, spinach.

  Benefits:
  - It is very important for development of skeleton, muscle contractions, bone and teeth formation, enzyme and hormone functioning.
  - Reduces the risk of pre-eclampsia.

- Help in growth of healthy heart, nerves and muscles.
- Improves blood clotting abilities.

- **Vitamin D**

  Source: Fish like salmon, dairy products, eggs, oranges, whole grain cereals, mushrooms, sun exposure at least 10-15minutes per day.

  Benefits:
  - Prevents preeclampsia.
  - Prevents gestational diabetes, pre-term, low birth babies.
  - Helps in maintain respiratory health of the babies.
  - Help in skeleton development and tooth enamel formation.

- **Vitamin C**

  Source: Citrus fruits like oranges, lemon, tomatoes, potatoes, broccoli.

  Benefits:
  - It is rich in anti-oxidants helps in preventing infections.
  - It helps in iron absorption.

- **Omega 3 fatty acid (DHA and EPA)**

  Sources: Salmon fish, chia seeds, flax seeds, walnuts, soya beans, green leafy vegetables like spinach, broccoli. You can also take protein powders which contains DHA.

Benefits:

- o Help in early development of baby's nervous system.
- o Develops cognitive thinking in babies and boosts memory.
- o Improves language skills, focus, attention span.
- o Reduces risk of pre-term labour.
- o Prevents asthma, blood pressure, allergies.
- o Improves circulation.
- o Reduces risk of ADHD and depression.

- **Iodine**: 50% more iodine required in pregnancy than normal.

    Sources: Yogurt, curd, milk, apple, iodized salt.

    Benefits:

    - o Helps in brain development.
    - o Helps in thyroid hormone synthesis in both mother and fetus.

- **Food to be avoided:** Avoid raw and partially cooked eggs to prevent salmonella food poisoning. Cook thoroughly until whites and yolk becomes solid.
    - o Avoid fish like tuna and shark because of high level of mercury, it can damage baby's developing nervous system.

- Avoid unpasteurized milk because it contains dangerous bacteria like salmonella, E.coli and listeria which can cause food poisoning.
- Avoid food and drinks rich in fats and sugar like soft drinks, chocolates, ice creams and fried foods etc. because they do not have any nutritional value. They can cause tooth decay, weight gain. Eating too much saturated fat can increase cholesterol amount in the body. Try to take unsaturated fats like olive oil, coconut oil etc.
- Avoid taking high amount of caffeine because it can result into low weight babies. Caffeine is present in coffees, tea, chocolates, soft drinks.
- Avoid smoking and alcohol these can cause growth restriction and low weight babies.

- **Exercise**: It forms one important component during antenatal period.
  - Moving your body is very important because it has many benefits specially in pregnancy like prevent excessive weight gain, pain reduction, boosts mood.
  - Help in digestion and prevents constipation.
  - Help in back ache.
  - Decrease risk of gestational diabetes and pre-eclampsia and caesarean section.
  - Strengthen your heart and blood vessels.
  - Exercise does not increase risk of miscarriage or early delivery.

- **When to start exercising**
  ◊ Meet your gynecologist before starting any type of exercise.
  ◊ Ideal time to start exercising is in second trimester because it is safe period. But you can do light exercise like walking, pelvic floor exercise or yoga in first trimester.
  ◊ In second and third trimester you can do brisk walking, yoga and swimming.
  ◊ You can do 150 minutes of moderate-intensity aerobics activity every week which includes brisk walking.
  ◊ You can divide the 150 minutes into 30-minute workouts on 5 days of the week or into smaller 10-minutes workouts throughout each day. You can go for three 10 minutes walks each day.
  ◊ You can do yoga poses like butterfly pose, thunderbolt pose (vajrasana), cow pose, legs up on the wall pose, sukhasana etc. These yoga works on three-dimensional mind, body and soul.
  ◊ Butterfly pose help in smooth delivery and relieves pain.
  ◊ Thunderbolt pose(vajrasana) helps in relieving backache and helps in digestion.
  ◊ Cow pose keeps the spine flexible, tones abdominal muscle and improves blood circulation.

- ◊ Leg up on the wall position relieves backache, increase blood flow to the pelvic area, ease swollen ankle and varicose vein.
- ◊ Sukhasana boosts mood, improves breathing and improves digestion.

Butterfly pose

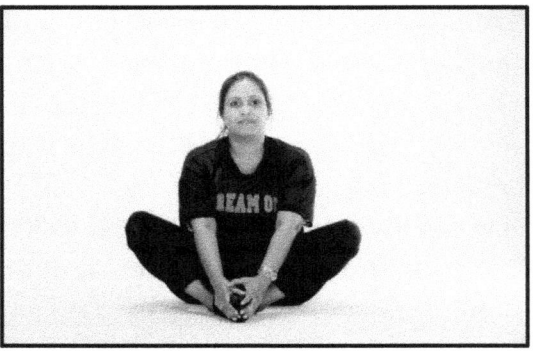

Thunderbolt pose(vajrasana)and leg up on the wall position

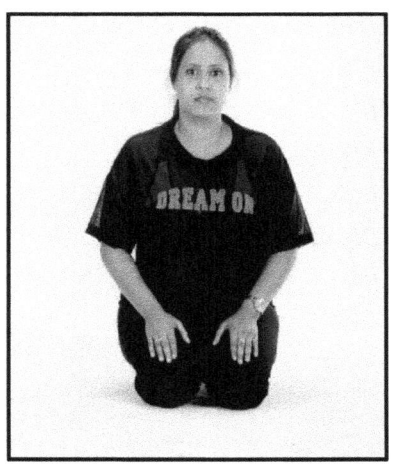

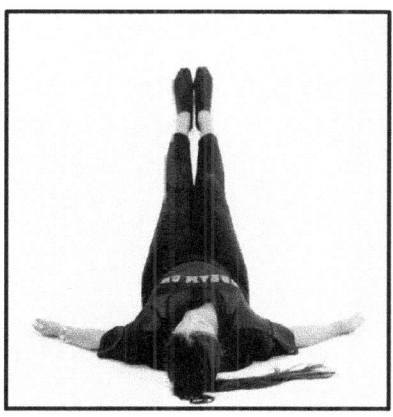

- **When you should avoid exercise?**
  ◊ When you are suffering from heart diseases.
  ◊ If your placenta is low lying (placenta previa).
  ◊ If you had history of pre-term birth.
  ◊ If you have short cervix and you have got stitches in your cervix.
  ◊ If you are carrying twins or triplets.
  ◊ If you are suffering from severe anemia or pre-eclampsia.

- **Weight gain in each trimester**
  o 1st trimester- 1kg
  o 2nd trimester- 5kg
  o 3rd trimester- 5 kg

Approximately 11 kg should be the weight gain in pregnancy not more than that.

- **Music therapy**

Music therapy during pregnancy is a complementary approach that utilizes music and its various elements to promote physical, emotional, and psychological well-being for expectant mothers. It can have several potential benefits to you and your baby.

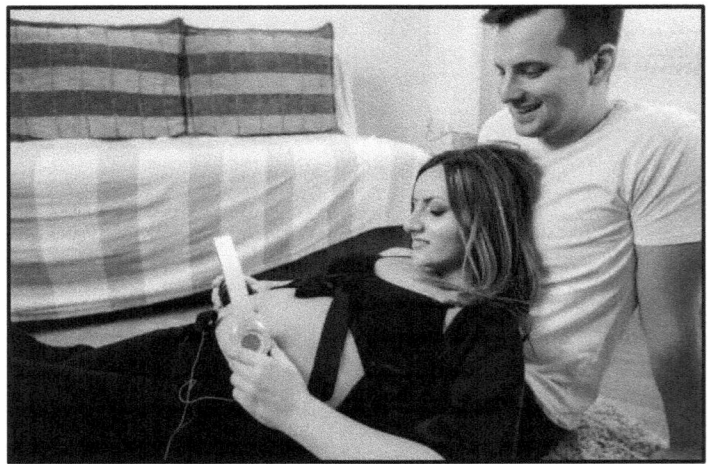

Here are some ways in which music therapy can be beneficial during your pregnancy:

- **Stress Reduction:** Pregnancy can be a stressful time due to physical discomfort and anxiety about labor and motherhood. Music can help reduce stress and promote relaxation. Slow, soothing music can lower cortisol levels, which are associated with stress.
- **Pain Management:** Music therapy can be used as a distraction technique during labor and childbirth. Listening to music can help women

focus on something other than pain and discomfort, making the experience more manageable.
- **Bonding:** Playing music or singing to the baby in the womb can help mothers and their partners feel a deeper connection with the baby before birth. The baby may also respond to the music by moving or kicking.
- **Emotional Expression:** Pregnancy often brings about a range of emotions. Music therapy can provide an outlet for emotional expression and can be a tool for coping with these feelings.
- **Improved Sleep:** Many pregnant women experience sleep disturbances. Listening to calming music before bedtime can promote better sleep quality.
- **Hormonal Balance:** Music can stimulate the release of endorphins, which are natural mood elevators. This can help balance hormones and improve mood during pregnancy.
- **Cognitive Development:** Some studies suggest that playing classical music to the baby in the womb may have a positive impact on the baby's cognitive development, although these findings are still debated.

- **When considering music therapy during pregnancy:**
  - **Consult with a healthcare provider:** Always discuss your plans for music therapy with your healthcare provider to ensure it's safe for your

specific situation. They can also provide guidance on any precautions or limitations.
- **Choose appropriate music:** Opt for music that is calming and soothing rather than overly stimulating. Classical music, soft instrumental music, or nature sounds are often good choices.
- **Be mindful of volume:** Keep the volume at a moderate level to protect the baby's developing ears. Loud music can be harmful.
- **Personal preference matters:** What is relaxing and enjoyable varies from person to person, so choose music that resonates with you and your partner.
- **Combine with other relaxation techniques:** Music therapy can complement other relaxation techniques such as prenatal yoga, meditation, and deep breathing exercises.

Remember that music therapy is not a replacement for medical care during pregnancy. It should be used as a supportive measure to enhance your overall well-being and reduce stress during this important time.

- **Meditation**
  - Stress in pregnancy like work stress, physical stress and hormonal stress and anxiety about labour pain can affect your baby's development. It has negative effect on immune system of the baby causing infection, digestive problems and respiratory problems.

- Long term untreated stress can lead to gestational diabetes, heart issues and pre-eclampsia etc.
- Anxiety releases stress hormones like cortisol, epinephrine and norepinephrine that can constrict blood vessels and reduce oxygen to the uterus and can affect growth of the baby.
- Meditation is the best tool to overcome stress and keep yourself calm throughout pregnancy and post pregnancy.
- Meditation reduces cortisol level and boosts endorphins and triggers body's relaxation response which includes low BP, heart rate, respiratory rate and make your body relax, decreases pain during labour, improves sleep.
- You can do meditation every day at least for 10 minutes.
- Sit in a quiet place and close your eyes and focus on your breath. It is very simple.

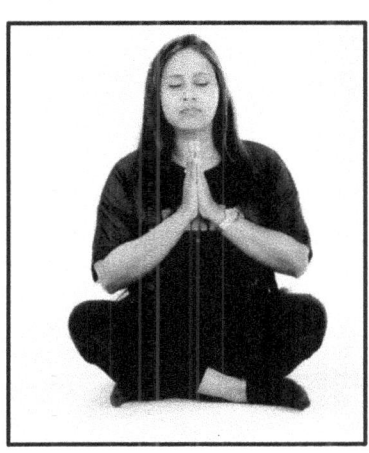

"A strong intention, a relaxed body and an open mind are the main ingredients for an active birth."

– Janet Balaskas

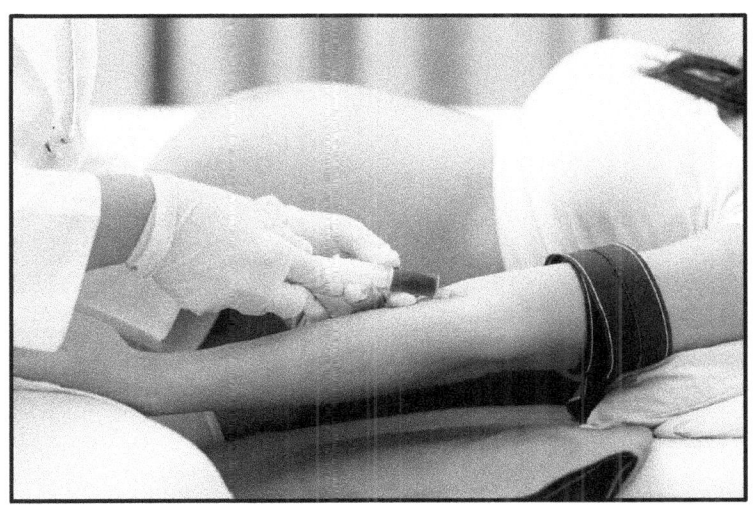

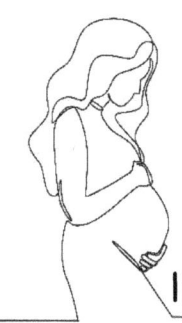

INVESTIGATIONS IN PREGNANCY

Investigations, also known as prenatal testing or prenatal screening, are an essential part of prenatal care during pregnancy. They are conducted to monitor the health of yours and your baby. These investigations serve several purposes as mentioned below.

- Monitoring the progress of your pregnancy.
- Assess your baby's health like growth and development, detection of potential abnormalities, congenital anomalies or genetic disorders.
- Identify your health concerns like anemia, gestational diabetes, thyroid disorders or infections.
- Risk assessment of you developing any medical disorder or genetic disorder or chromosomal abnormalities in baby.
- Prevention and management of complications or conditions that arise during pregnancy.

- Emotional support to you and your husband by confirming the well-being of your baby and ruling out potential concerns.

Commonly performed investigations

The specific investigations can vary based on factors such as your age, medical history, family history and circumstances. Here are some common investigations done during pregnancy and their justifications.

- **Blood tests**: Blood tests are routinely conducted during pregnancy to assess various aspects of maternal health and screen for potential issues. These may include:
  o **Blood Group and Rh Typing**: Determines the mother's blood type and Rh factor. It helps identify if the mother is Rh-negative and requires Rh immune globulin to prevent complications.
  o **Complete Blood Count (CBC):** Checks for anemia or other blood disorders that can affect the mother's health and the baby's oxygen supply.
  o **Blood Glucose Tests**: Screens for gestational diabetes, a condition that can develop during pregnancy and affect both the mother and the baby.
  o **Sexually Transmitted Infection (STI) Testing**: Identifies STIs such as syphilis, HIV, hepatitis B, and others, which can potentially affect the baby during pregnancy or delivery.

- **Urine Tests:** Urine tests are performed to check for various health markers and detect potential issues, including:
    o **Urine Analysis:** Screens for conditions such as urinary tract infections, proteinuria (excessive protein in urine), or signs of kidney problems.
    o **Urine Culture:** Detects the presence of bacteria in the urinary tract, which can cause urinary tract infections and potentially harm the pregnancy.
- **Ultrasound Scans:** Ultrasound scans use sound waves to create images of the baby and the reproductive organs. They are performed at various stages of pregnancy for different reasons, including:
    o **Dating Ultrasound (6-10 weeks):** Determines the gestational age and estimated due date of the baby, number of fetuses, pregnancy location whether it is in uterus, tube or anywhere else.

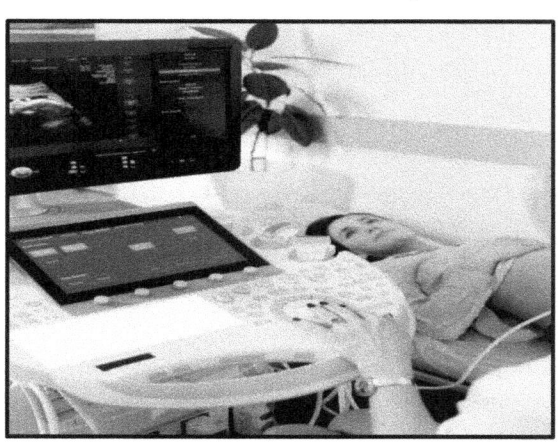

- **Nuchal Translucency (NT) Scan (12-14 weeks):** Screens for chromosomal abnormalities, particularly Down's syndrome, by measuring the fluid accumulation at the back of the baby's neck.
- **Anomaly Scan (18-22 weeks):** Evaluates the baby's anatomy and looks for any structural abnormalities or birth defects.
- **Fetal Echo:** It is done along with anomaly scan when there is any heart anomaly or any medical condition like diabetes etc. It is done between 18-25th weeks.
- **Growth Ultrasounds (28-32 weeks):** Monitors the baby's growth, amniotic fluid levels, and placenta function throughout pregnancy. Sometimes it is done along with doppler study to look for blood flow in the fetus.

- **Genetic Screening and Testing:** These investigations are offered to assess the risk of genetic disorders in the baby, based on factors such as maternal age, family history, or specific indications. They may include:
  - **Carrier Screening:** Identifies if the parents carry genes for certain genetic conditions, such as cystic fibrosis or sickle cell anemia.
  - **Non-Invasive Prenatal Testing (NIPT):** Screens for common chromosomal abnormalities, including Down syndrome, using a blood sample from the mother

- o **Diagnostic Testing:** Invasive procedures, such as chorionic villus sampling (CVS) or amniocentesis, are performed to diagnose or rule out specific genetic disorders or chromosomal abnormalities.
- **Group B Streptococcus (GBS) Screening:** GBS is a bacterium that some women carry without symptoms, but it can cause infections in new born. Testing is done around the 35th to 37th week of pregnancy to identify if you are having GBS or not and to determine if antibiotics during labour are necessary to prevent transmission to your baby.
- **Additional Investigations:** Depending on your condition, your doctor may recommend additional investigations, such as fetal echocardiography (to assess the baby's heart), doppler and biophysical profile (to evaluate the baby's well-being), or specific tests to monitor or diagnose any maternal or fetal health concerns.

It's important to remember that the necessity and timing of these investigations vary based on individual factors and the associated condition.

"The role of science should be to investigate the unexplained, not explain the uninvestigated."
— Stephen Rorke

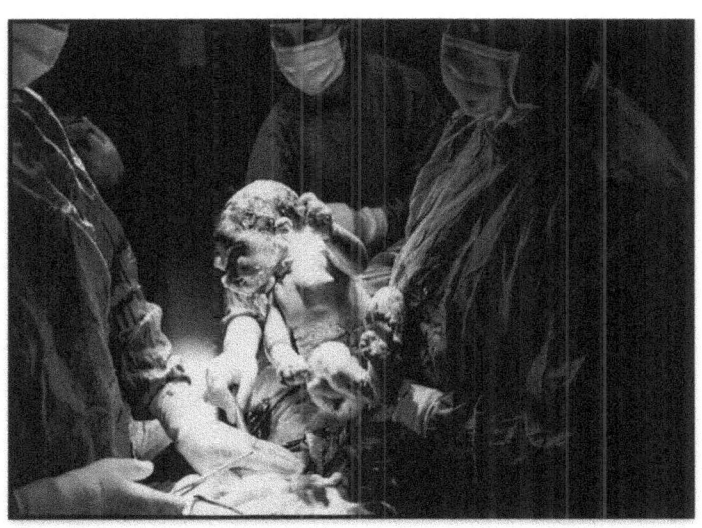

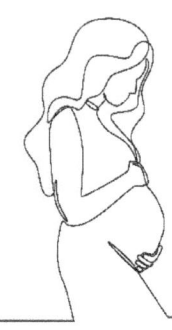

LABOUR, DELIVERY AND POST DELIVERY CARE

Labour and delivery follow a pattern like starting of contraction then softening and opening of cervix, rupture of amniotic sac, contractions become stronger and stronger followed by delivery.

- **Signs of labour:**
  - **Painful uterine contractions:** You will feel lower abdominal pain radiating to back and thigh with increase in intensity at regular interval with relaxation between. It won't stop with painkillers and your contraction will become more stronger as labour will progress.
  - **Show:** It is blood mixed with mucus .
  - **Rupture of water bag:** Your water bag may break.
- **Induction of labour**

  Some women even after 40 weeks also do not get labour pain spontaneously or your pregnancy need to be terminated earlier or at 38 weeks due to medical issue like hypertension, gestational diabetes. In those conditions your doctor may use some methods to initiate labour pain and that is known as induction of labour. In other words, "Induction of labour" is nothing but artificial initiation of your labour pain. There are various methods of induction but mainly three are used.

- **Foley's catheter:** It is a tube which is inserted intra cervically, and inflated with 60ml of normal saline and foley's is tied to the maternal thigh. It is removed after 12 hours and some hospitals it is left and it expels on its own. It helps in shorting, softening and dilation of cervix.
- **Prostaglandin gel:** It is a gel which is kept intra cervically and left for 6 hours, maximum three doses every six hourly. It helps in ripening and dilation of cervix.
- **Misoprostol:** It is a tablet, which is kept intravaginally or given orally maximum 3 doses 6th hourly or 4th hourly. It helps in ripening and dilation of cervix.
- **Castor oil** is also used by some gynecologist for cervical ripening and dilation as well. When patient reaches term then she is asked to take 15 to 60 ml castor oil in juice in the night.
- **Sweeping of membranes:** In this your doctor will do internal examination and will sweep out membranes from the lower uterine segment. It helps in release of prostaglandin which helps in induction of labour.

- o **Artificial rupture of membranes (breaking the water):** In this your water bag is broken by your doctor. This also helps in release of prostaglandins which induces labour.
- **Painless delivery (labour analgesia):** Labour is very stressful and painful situation. So let's talk about measures for painless delivery. There are many options now which can help to reduce your labour pain and reduce your anxiety.
  - o **Non-medical methods**
    - **Deep breathing exercise:** Just 're-lax', stay calm and breathe deeply. Conscious breathing activates parasympathetic system and shuts off sympathetic system, reduces your heart rate and blood pressure. It involves inhale and exhale which stimulates the parasympathetic nervous system, leading to increased blood supply and oxygenation. It releases of endorphins which decreases heart rate and makes you calm. Endorphins suppress the sympathetic nervous system resulting in decreased release of stress hormone cortisol. It helps reducing the perception of your labour pain as well as in shortening the duration of second stage of labour. So just try to relax and breathe deeply.
    - **Hydrotherapy (water birth):** Immerse yourself in water or you can take shower with warm water. It helps in decreasing pain and anxiety and it gives relaxation. It reduces pressure on

the spine, helps the pelvis to open up and cervical dilation. It decreases augmentation of labour, decreases risk of cesarean section and use of epidural analgesia.

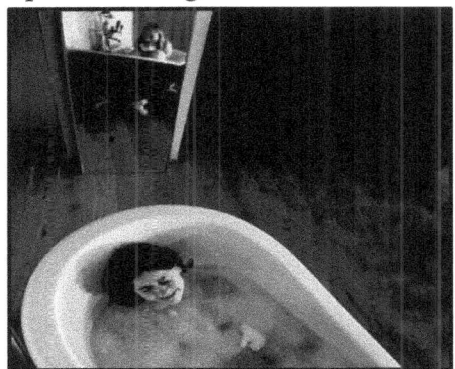

- **Move, walk or change position:** Move, walk or change positions, it helps in pain reduction and changing position frequently moves the bones of pelvis, helping the baby to descend.
- **Touch and massage:** Gives relaxation and reduces pain.
- **Acupuncture and acupressure:** Helps in pain reduction.
- **Aromatherapy:** Using highly concentrated essential oils can help in pain reduction.
- **Hot and cold fomentation:** Application of hot and cold is easy, inexpensive, require no prior practice and it helps in pain reduction too. You can apply heat on back, lower abdomen and genital area.

- o **Medical methods**
  - **Tramadol injection:** It is a synthetic analogue of codeine, a centrally acting synthetic analgesic/ painkiller given in case of excruciating pain. But, previously it was thought that it causes neonatal respiratory depression. But, recent studies says that it does not exert inhibitory effects on the respiratory center, means it does not causes respiratory problems in newborn. Once you are in active stage of labour (means your cervix is more than 4cm dilated). Injection Tramadol is given intra-muscularly 100mg single dose. Other injections like Pethidine or Diamorphine can also help in pain reduction.

    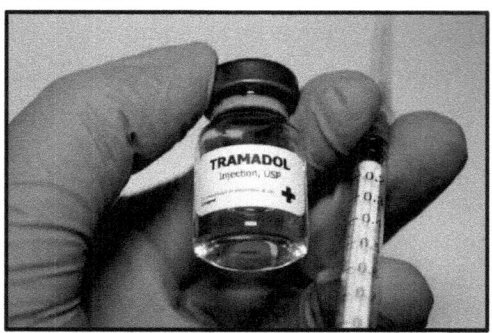

  - **ENTONOX (inhalation of Gas for pain relief):** It is mixer of nitrous oxide gas (laughing gas) and oxygen. It helps in pain reduction. It is safe for you and baby too. A mask is connected to the oxygen cylinder, you have keep that mask on your nose and mouth during contractions and breath deeply. It takes 15-20 seconds to work. It can be used at any stage of labour.

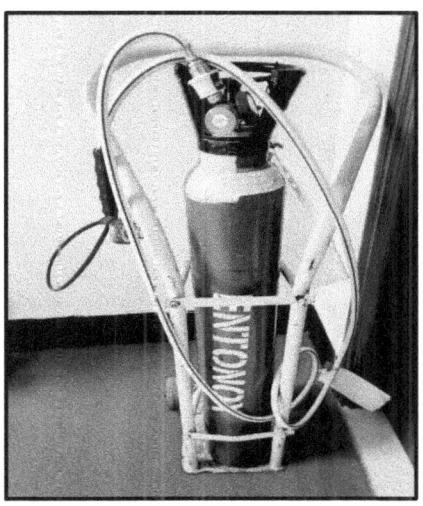

- **Epidural analgesia:** In this medicine is injected in to the epidural space of spinal cord by your anesthesiologist. It makes lower body numb from umbilicus to legs. But you will feel pressure in second stage so that you will be able to push the baby. It is safe for mother and the baby. It does not interfere with the progress of the labour and delivery.

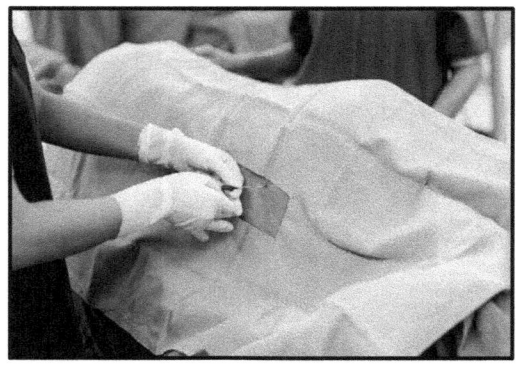

- **TENS:** (Transcutaneous electrical nerve stimulation)- It is a hand-held device with electrodes and it emits low voltage current. Electrodes are placed on the back and low voltage current transmit through the nerves to the spinal cord. That reduces the transmission of pain signal to the spinal cord and brain and help in pain reduction.

Let's talk about stages of labour.

- **Stages of labour**

There are four stages of labour:

- **Stage 1:** It starts from commencement of true labour. pain to full dilatation of cervix (means your cervix opens up to 10 cm). Your doctor will do internal examination every 4-6 hourly to check your cervical dilatation.
- **Stage 2:** It starts from full dilatation of cervix to delivery of your baby.

- o **Stage 3:** It starts from delivery of your baby to expulsion of placenta
- o **Stage 4:** In this stage you are observed for 1 hour for excessive bleeding and vitals monitoring.

- **What you need to do during labour**
  - o Keep yourself calm and breathe deeply.
  - o Keep yourself hydrated.
  - o When your cervix is fully dilated, your doctor will shift you to the labour board ask you to push while contractions. So, push during contractions and relax and rest when you don't have contraction. You can sip water when you are resting.
  - o When your baby's head is seen, your doctor will give local anesthesia followed by episiotomy and then deliver your baby.

But there are some conditions in which normal delivery is risky so your doctor will suggest you for cesarean section. I have listed some conditions below:

- o If your baby's heartbeat is dropping (fetal distress)
- o If your placenta is low lying (Placenta previa)
- o If your baby's presentation is breech or transverse
- o If your pelvic bone smaller for your baby (cephalic pelvic disproportion)
- o If your baby has passed stools in the womb

- Previous history of cesarean section (trial of labour is given only if ICU facilities and expert doctor's team are available in the hospital).

- **Caesarean section**

    For cesarean section are of two types, one which is done in emergency and second which is done electively. For elective cesarean section, your doctor will ask you to fast for 6-12hours. Under spinal/general anesthesia, your baby is delivered by opening your abdominal layers.

- **Post-partum bleeding/ hemorrhage (PPH)**

    It is very serious complication following delivery. It can happen to anyone, but it is more common in women who have given birth 2-3 times, women with overdistended abdomen in case high liquor level or twins or in case preeclampsia or in a woman who had prolonged labour etc. When you lose more than 500ml of blood in normal delivery and 1 liter of blood in cesarean section , it is diagnosed as PPH. It needs emergency attention. You need to call your doctor immediately. But some remedies I will suggest here. If you anticipate PPH then start feeding your baby, this will help in release of oxytocin which will help in contraction of uterus and second, elevate your legs and put your head down towards your back this will reduce the blood flow towards your pelvic area.

- **Post-delivery care**
    o You must continue to take balanced diet as advised by your doctor or other health care professional.
    o Take plenty of water and milk
    o Wound care is very important following delivery. It depends on your mode of delivery i.e., perineal wound in case of vaginal birth or abdominal wound in case of caesarean birth. In both keep the wound dry and clean.
    o Apply antiseptic cream as advised by your doctor.
    o Take bath daily and clean the wound with soap.
    o Avoid lifting heavy weight.
    o Breast care: Clean your nipple before and after breast-feeding.
    o Avoid intercourse for 6 weeks.
- **Common aliments following delivery**
    o **Contractions:** You will feel mild contractions after delivery on and off like menstrual cramps. This is known as after pain. It prevents excessive bleeding by compressing the uterine vessels. It is common during breastfeeding because of release of oxytocin hormone. You don't need to worry about it much.
    o **Tender breasts/engorgement:** Wear tight breast support, hot fomentation followed by expressing the milk, you can keep cold cabbage leaves under breast support and don't cover

nipples. It will help in relieving pain. When pain is severe or in case of fever, consult your doctor.

- **Sore nipple:** Make sure your baby latches on to your breast correctly. The baby's mouth should be opened very wide and your entire areola should be in the baby's mouth. You can let milk dry on your nipples. This dried milk can protect the skin on your nipple. Don't use alcohol, soap, or scented cleansers on your breasts. These can cause the nipples to dry and crack. Don't wear nursing pads that are lined with plastic. They hold in moisture and can cause chapping. If you have cracked or bleeding nipples, consult your healthcare provider or a lactation consultant. They will make sure that your baby's latch is correct and may suggest topical treatment, like pure lanolin. With the advice of your doctor you may use nipple shield.

- **Hair loss:** During pregnancy, estrogen hormone is high which makes your hair grow and once you deliver, estrogen drops and your hair starts falling. But its temporary, by your child's first birthday your hair fall problem will reduce. Eat healthy and avoid tight ponytails.

- **Mood swings/ postpartum baby blues**: It can last from few days to weeks. You may feel confused and lost, having sleep problem. Don't neglect these symptoms and consult your doctor.

- **Lactation failure:** Its very common problem after delivery. Try to be stress free because stress releases cortisol which inhibits prolactin hormone, hence reduces your milk production. Detail is discussed in the chapter lactation.

With every new born baby, a little sun rises."

- Irmgard Erath

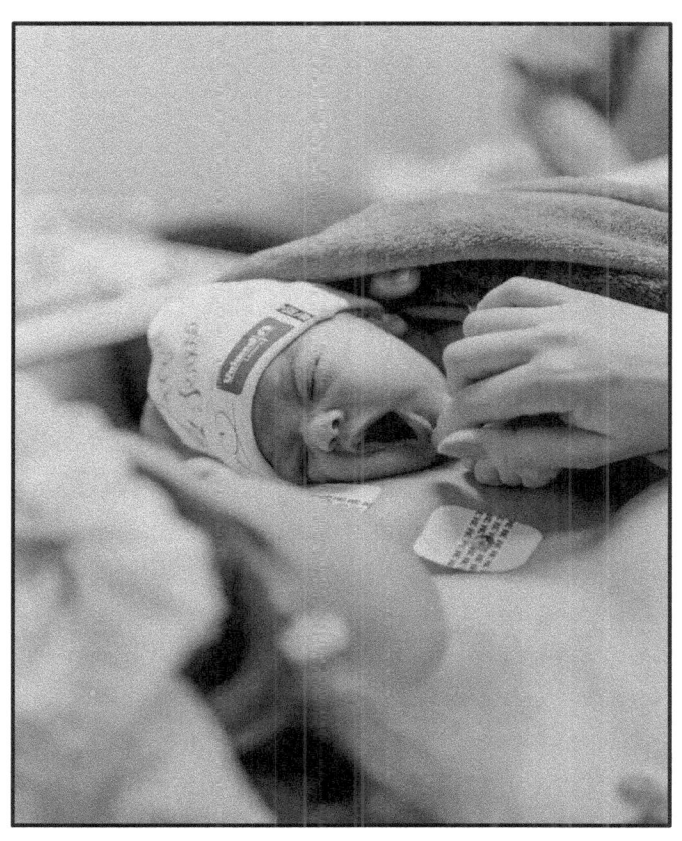

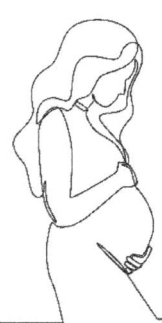

NEWBORN CARE

Meeting your baby and getting to your baby must be very exciting for you. But, you must be tired and in pain, needing adequate rest. Here we will discuss how you can take care of your newborn.

- **Breastfeeding**: Breastfeeding has many benefits for your baby. First few days you will get colostrum also known as "liquid gold" because it is thick and yellow in color. It is rich in nutrition, antibodies and anti-oxidants. It changes to normal milk after few days. Start breastfeeding withing an hour after giving birth and continue exclusively till 6 months and with solids till 2 years. Avoid cow milk because it can cause intestinal issues. Details is being maintained in chapter 'Lactation'.
- **Cord care:** After birth, the doctor will cut and clamp the cord and leave a small bit of it. You need to keep the cord clean and dry. It will drop off after few days spontaneously. In case of bleeding or discharge, show your baby to the doctor.
- **Diapering**: You can use cotton cloth or diaper for your baby, both are safe. Change it frequently to

avoid infection, pneumonia and rashes. If baby develops rashes or to prevent it apply thick layer of diaper rash cream containing zinc oxide to create thick barrier on the skin on genital and anal area. You can use petroleum jelly as well.
- **Prevent hypothermia:** Maintaining a warm environment is very important especially newborn because they are more vulnerable for temperature changes. Make sure baby's head is covered, hands and feet are covered. One rule you can follow add one more layer to the baby what you are comfortable wearing in the same environment.
- Avoid putting kajal, scented powder, honey in the mouth or vigorous massage etc.
- **Jaundice**: It is yellow discoloration of newborn's skin and eyes. It occurs because the baby's blood contains excess of bilirubin and baby's liver is too immature to get rid of bilirubin in the blood. Generally, occurs 2nd to 4th day of birth and disappears within 10 days. To check infant jaundice, gently press baby's forehead or nose, if skin looks yellow then it is a mild jaundice. Adequate feeding can prevent infant jaundice so feed you baby 8-12 times for first few days. Medical attention required in case of severe jaundice.
- **Fontanelle**: It is a diamond shaped space 'soft spot' on the top of the head and back. They are for development of the brain. Front soft spot closes around 18 months and back soft spot closes at 2-3 months. Avoid touching if frequently.

Conception to confinement

- **Oiling**: Massage makes baby calm, enhances sleep and tone of the body, strengthens bones. But, you should avoid oiling until one month after birth. You can use mustard or coconut oil for massage. While massaging abdomen, rub your fingers in clock wise direction because it prevents from gas development and abdominal issues. Be gentle!
- **Bathing and skin care:** It is your choice how frequently you want to give bath to the baby. Warm bath makes babies calm and help them sleep. Use gentle body wash or soap and shampoo with no fragrance for bath because baby's skin is sensitive and delicate and developing state. Apply baby's moisturizer twice daily after bath and before sleeping in the night for healthy skin. Avoid using adult skin care products!
- **Sleeping**: Newborn babies sleep around 14-17 hours in 24 hours. Make sure you use firm surface for sleeping your baby and warm blanket to cover. Don't use pillow because they may feel suffocating.
- **Crying**: All babies cry. For three months babies cry more. When baby is crying, check that nappy is wet or baby is hungry, sick, uncomfortable or in pain. Talk or sing, feed, change the nappy or move the baby or go for a walk with baby and if cry gets too much, take medical help.
- **Vaccination:** BCG to prevent tuberculosis, Hepatitis B for prevention of Hepatitis B and OPV to prevent polio are given at birth. Rest vaccines are

given according to National Immunization Schedule.

Care of Preterm/ Premature Babies

o   Premature babies or low birth babies need extra care and support, warmth, protection from infections, safety and love.
o   Kangaroo mother care is best for premature babies for warmth and weight gain. It is a technique by which premature babies are held on an adult's chest for skin-to-skin contact. Babies are placed on mother's/ father's chest and stays there wrapped in a cloth tied at the mother's back.

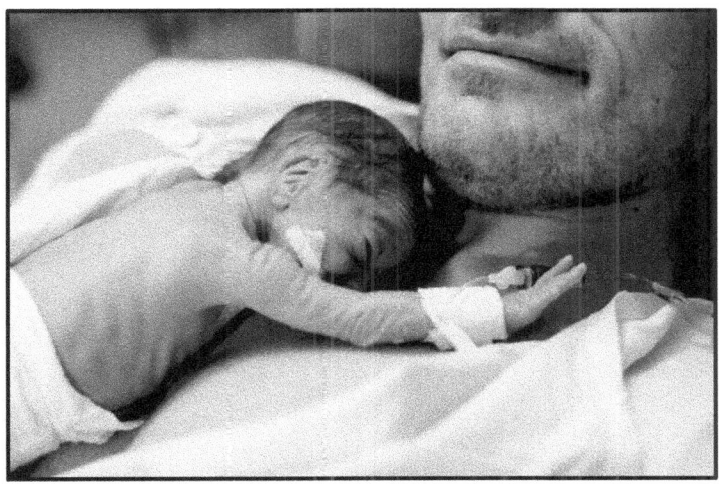

Giving birth is not a matter of pushing, expelling the baby, but of yielding, surrendering to birth energy."

— Marie Reid

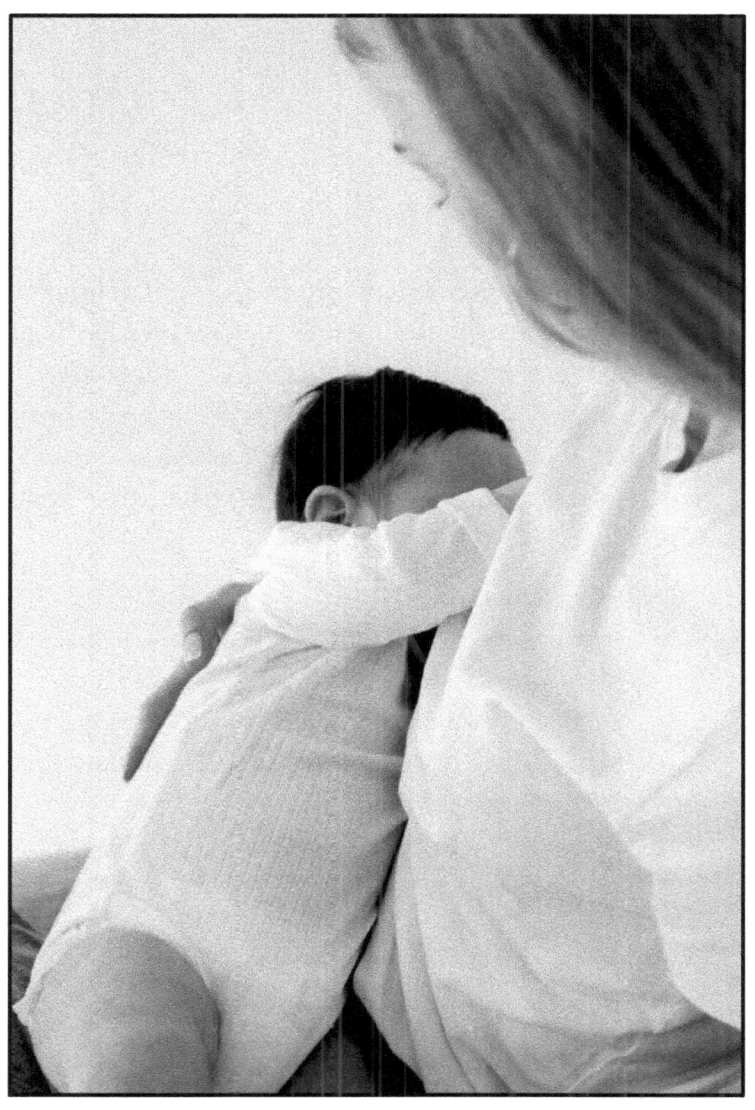

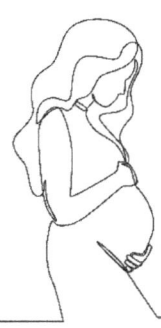

LACTATION

Lactation is the process of producing and releasing milk from the mammary glands in your breasts. This process is essential for establishment of successful breast feeding. It begins during pregnancy in response to hormonal change. This change prepares mammary glands to make milk in preparation for the birth of your baby.

- **Process of lactation**
    - It involves two stages i.e., secretory initiation and secretory activation
    - Secretory initiation takes place during the second half of pregnancy with small amounts of milk in the form of colostrum.
    - Secretory activation starts with copious milk production after delivery.
- **Benefit of lactation**
    - **Benefit for your Baby:**
    - **Optimal nutrition:** Breast milk is highly nutritious and provides all the essential nutrients, vitamins and minerals that your

baby needs for healthy growth and development. It contains the perfect balance of proteins, fats and carbohydrates for your baby's growing body.

- **Immune protection:** Breast milk contains antibodies and immune factors that help protect your baby against infections, allergies and illness. It boosts your baby's immune system and lowers the risk of respiratory infections, ear infections, gastrointestinal infections etc.
- **Digestive health:** Breast milk is easily digested by your baby's immature digestive system, reducing the risk of constipation, diarrhea and digestive discomfort.
- **Cognitive development:** Research suggests that breastfeeding may contribute to improved cognitive development and higher IQ scores later in life.
- **Bonding and emotional connection:** Breast feeding promotes bonding and emotional attachment between you and your baby. The skin-to-skin contact and close physical proximity during breastfeeding also help in creating a strong emotional connection.
- **Benefit for you:**
  - **Bonding and emotional wellbeing:** Lactation promotes the release of oxytocin, a hormone that promotes bonding and feelings of

relaxation and well-being in you. It can enhance your emotional connection with your baby and provide a sense of fulfilment.
- **Postpartum recovery:** Lactation stimulates the uterus to contact, which helps its return to its pre-pregnancy size more quickly. It may also help with postpartum weight loss by burning calories.
- **Reduce risk of chronic health conditions:** Lactation has been associated with a lower risk of certain health conditions for the you, including breast and ovarian cancer, type 2 diabetes and postpartum depression.
- **Convenience and cost savings:** Breast milk always available and at the right temperature, eliminating the need for formula preparation and sterilization of the bottle. This convenience can save time and money.
- **Environmental benefits:** Breastfeeding is environmentally friendly, as it avoids the production, packaging and waste associated with formula feeding.

- **Factors initiating or establishing lactation**
  - Put your baby to breast following delivery, vaginal or LSCS, at the earliest.
  - Regular removal of milk and stimulation of the nipple in the form of breast feeding.

- o This triggers prolactin release from the anterior pituitary gland and oxytocin from the posterior pituitary gland.
- o Prolactin helps in synthesis of milk and oxytocin helps in ejection of milk

- **Factors increasing lactation**
  - o **Frequent and effective breastfeeding /pumping:** The more you stimulate your breast, the more milk your body is likely to produce. Breastfeed or pump frequently, ideally every 2-3 hours. Ensure your baby is latching correctly, and if using breast pump, choose one that suits you and use it according to the manufacture's instruction.
  - o **Empty the breast:** Make sure to fully empty your breasts during each feeding or pumping session. This helps signal your body to produce more milk. If your baby is not able to feed effectively, you can use a breast pump to empty the breasts after nursing
  - o **Stay hydrated:** drinking an adequate amount of water is important for milk production. Aim for at least 8 cups of water or other healthy fluids per day.

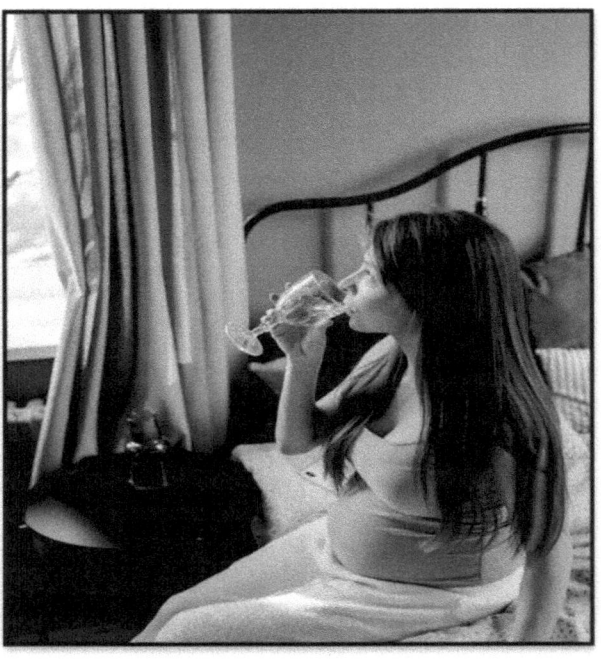

- **Proper nutrition:** Consuming a well-balanced diet is crucial for overall health and lactation. Include foods rich in nutrients such as protein, calcium, iron, and healthy fats. Oatmeal, leafy greens, salmon, whole grains, and legumes are often recommended for breastfeeding mothers.
- **Rest and relaxation:** Stress and exhaustion can negatively impact milk supply. Ensure you are getting enough rest and try to manage stress through relaxation techniques like deep breathing exercise, mediation or gentle exercise.

- o **Skin-to-skin contact:** Holding your baby skin-to-skin can stimulate hormone production and enhance the breast-feeding relationship. This practice also helps regulate the baby's body temperature and encourages bonding.
- o **Seek support:** reach out to a lactation consultant, a breast-feeding support group or a health care professional experienced in lactation for guidance and assistance. They can provide personalized advice and support to address any specific concerns you may have.

- **Lactation failure**

  Lactation failure, also known as insufficient milk supply or low milk production, occurs when you unable to produce an adequate amount of breast milk to meet her baby's nutritional needs. It can be a temporary or ongoing condition and can happen for various reasons. Common factors are as follows:

  - o **Hormonal issues:** Hormonal imbalances or certain medical conditions, such as polycystic ovary syndrome (PCOS), thyroid disorders, or hormonal medications, can interfere with milk production.
  - o **Ineffective breastfeeding technique:** If your baby is not latching properly or not nursing frequently or effectively, it can impact milk supply. An improper latch or inefficient sucking can hinder milk transfer and reduce

stimulation to the breast, leading to decreased milk production.
- **Insufficient breast tissue:** If you have less glandular tissue in their breast, it can affect their milk-making capacity.
- **Medical conditions and medication:** Certain medical conditions, such as breast surgery resulting reduced breast tissue can affect milk production. Additionally, specific medications, including some hormonal contraceptives or decongestants, may suppress milk supply.
- **Stress and emotional factors:** High levels of stress, anxiety or emotional distress can interfere with the let-down reflex and milk production. It's important to create a calm and supportive environment for breastfeeding.
- **Previous breastfeeding difficulties:** Women who have had challenges with breastfeeding in previous experience may be more prone to lactation failure in subsequent pregnancies.

- **Strategies to manage lactation failure**

  If you face this situation, you may try following tips:
  - Increase breastfeeding frequency.
  - Ensure proper latching.
  - Use of breast compression technique (Breast pump or hand expression).

o If above methods fail ensure the baby's nutritional needs supplements with either Donor or formula milk.

- **Storage of breast milk**

  You can store your breast milk for your baby to be used as and when required. This is useful if you are working and looking for more flexibility. Before expressing or handling breast milk, wash your hands with soap and water. You can also use breast pump for collection of your breast milk.

  o **Container**: Then store the expressed milk in a clean, capped food-grade glass container or hard plastic container that's not made with the chemical bisphenol A (BPA). You can also use special plastic bags designed for milk collection and storage. Don't store breast milk in disposable bottle liners or plastic bags designed for general household use.

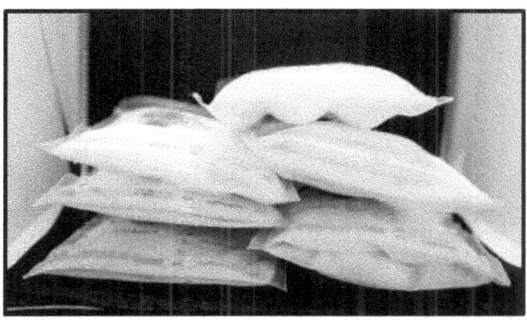

- **Storage**: Ensure to use waterproof labels and ink to label each container with the date you expressed the breast milk. If you're storing expressed milk at your baby's child care facility, add your baby's name to the label.

Place the containers in the back of the refrigerator or freezer, where the temperature is the coolest. If you don't have access to a refrigerator or freezer, store the milk temporarily in an insulated cooler with ice packs.

- **Duration of storage:** How long you can safely keep expressed breast milk depends on the storage method. Consider these general guidelines:
  - **Room temperature.** Up to six hours. However, it's optimal to use or properly store the breast milk within four hours, especially if the room is warm.
  - **Insulated cooler.** With ice packs for up to one day.
  - **Refrigerator.** Up to four days. However, it's optimal to use or freeze the milk within three days.
  - **Deep freezer:** Up to 12 months. However, using the frozen milk within six months is optimal.

Research suggests that the longer you store breast milk ,whether in the refrigerator or in the freezer , the greater the loss of vitamin C in the milk.

o **Use after storage**: Thaw the oldest milk first. Place the frozen container in the refrigerator the night before you intend to use it. You can also gently warm the milk by placing it under warm running water or in a bowl of warm water. Don't heat a frozen bottle in the microwave or very quickly on the stove. Some parts of the milk might be too hot, and others cold. Also, some research suggests that rapid heating can affect the milk's antibodies. Many experts recommend discarding thawed milk that isn't used within 24 hours.

A baby nursing at a mother's breast is an undeniable affirmation of our rootedness in nature.

- David Suzuki

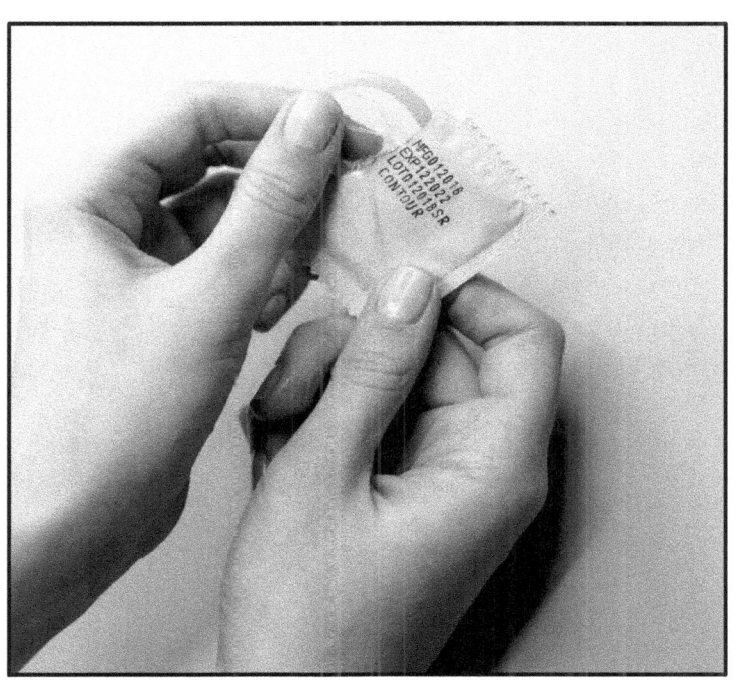

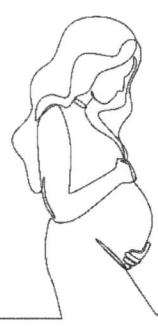

CONTRACEPTION AFTER DELIVERY

You may become pregnant by 4 weeks, if you are not breast feeding your baby or 6 weeks even if you are breast feeding if you don't take adequate precaution. You can have intercourse after 6 weeks of delivery. There are many options of contraception. I will list them below, you can consult your doctor and use them to prevent further pregnancy.

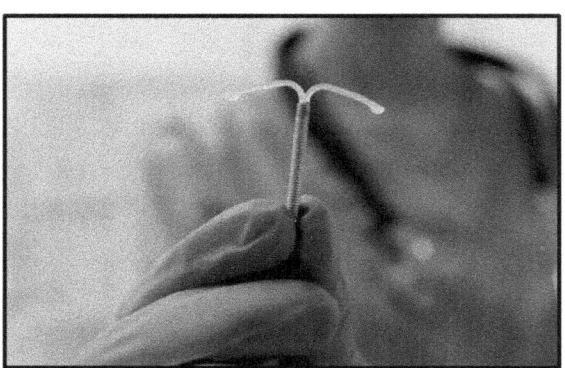

- **Intra Uterine Copper Device (IUCD)**: You can go for Cu-T insertion which protects you for 5 years (Cu IUCD 375) and 10 years (Cu IUCD 380). After delivery your doctor will insert it inside your uterus within 48 hours of delivery or after 6 weeks of delivery. It prevents sperm and egg from meeting and prevents implantation of fertilized egg. It can used by lactating mothers. Some patient's complaints of heavy bleeding after insertion. Yes, bleeding can occur for 2-3 months in some, but most of the times it settles down of its own. So, don't get panic or get it removed. When you suffer from heavy bleeding, meet your doctor for appropriate advice. This is not preferred in heart disease and diabetes patients because of increased chance of infection.

- **Progesterone only Pill (POP)**: You can use POP after delivery. It doesn't affect the lactation.
- **Injectable contraception**: Inj. DMPA(Antara), given in once every three months to prevent pregnancy. Usually you will not have menses in first year of use. There may be weight gain and delay in return to fertility of up to 1 year after discontinuation of the medicine.
- **Emergency contraceptive pills**- This pill can be taken within 72 hours of unprotected intercourse.
- **Oral combined contraceptive pill (OCP)**: it's not advisable to take immediately following delivery because it affects lactation. However, you can take low dose OC pills after 8 months of delivery and getting the period.
- **Tubal ligation**: If your family is complete the you can go for tubal ligation within seven days of delivery or after 6 months of delivery. In this

surgery your both fallopian tubes are cut and ligated.
- **Lactational amenorrhea method**: If you are feeding your baby properly, you may not get your period. This can be a temporary method of contraception. During this period, ovulation does not happen so pregnancy cannot happen.

God commanded his people to "Be fruitful and multiply," and contraception is seen as specifically flouting this instruction.

Unknown

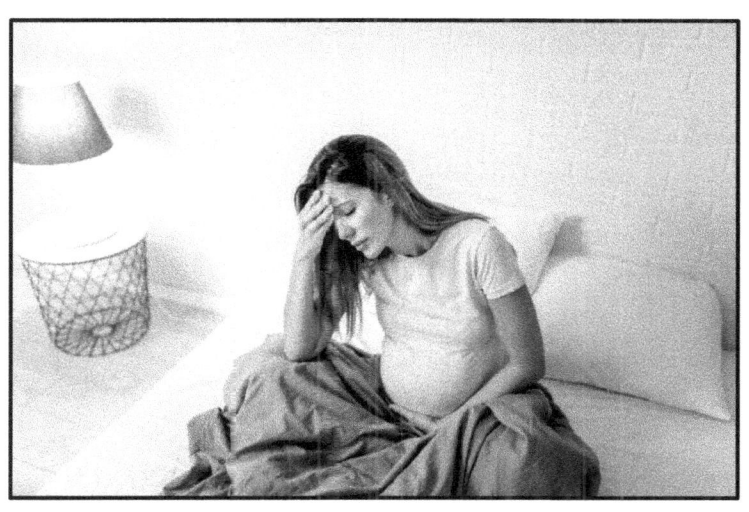

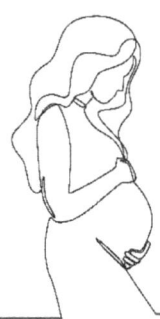

COMMON PROBLEMS IN PREGNANCY

You may face some common problems during pregnancy. Sometimes these problems reappear in subsequent pregnancy

- **Nausea and vomiting:** After embryo attaches to the uterus (implantation), your body starts producing HCG hormone. Estrogen hormones also rises in pregnancy leading nausea and vomiting. It starts usually before nine weeks and subsides after by 14 weeks. In some women it stays little longer and some women it stays throughout pregnancy. Take dry biscuits and toasts, take frequent small meals, you can take ginger when you feel nauseous. Meet your doctor when you get more than 4-5 episodes in a day.
- **Breast changes**: Your breasts will grow bigger and even tender. Areola also becomes more darker due to pigmentation. These changes are normal and happens a result of hormonal changes in pregnancy. Use tight breast support.
- **Stretch marks:** Its very common in pregnancy because of hormonal changes. It occurs due other

reasons also like if you are dehydrated or your skin is dry. But main reason for stretch marks is that your baby is growing and your belly is growing so skin get stretched. Your skin has elastic and non-elastic fibers and when your skin stretches, non-elastic fibers breaks. Elasticity varies from person to person and so in some women stretch marks are fewer and some have more. The best way to prevent it by applying moisturizer twice daily from the beginning of the pregnancy. You can use olive oil, coconut, almond oil, shea butter or cocoa butter. Keep yourself hydrated, do regular exercise so your muscle will be toned. Eat lots of citrus fruits like orange, lemon which will help in collagen production and makes your skin more elastic.

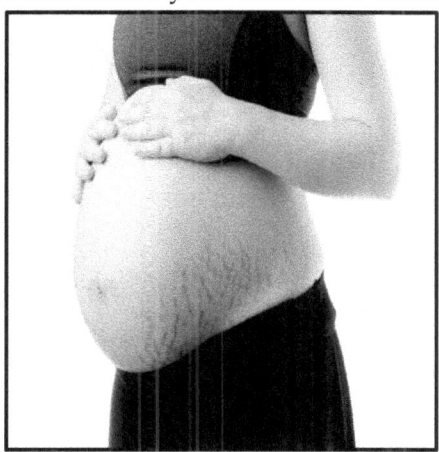

- **Nasal congestion**: Its very common in pregnancy because of "progesterone hormone", which causes mucous membrane and sinuses swells up causing nasal congestion. You can use

nasal saline nasal spray, hot shower or steam inhalation.
- **Constipation**: Due to "Progesterone Hormone" colon motility reduces and causes constipation. Your baby is also growing which causes pressure on the colon leading to constipation. Eat lots of fruits specially banana. You can take 1 table spoon of ghee or 3 table spoons of isabgol husk every day night. Drink plenty of oral fluids.
- **Backache**: It is very common problem in pregnancy. As pregnancy advances, your baby grows and abdominal muscles stretches and become weak putting more strain on your back and joints. Hormonal changes also relax the ligaments of the joints of pelvic to make it flexible for delivery and this causes backpain. Avoid high heels, sleep on firm bed, avoid lifting heavy weight. Hot water bags or ice packs can soothe your sore muscle. Sit in correct posture.
- **Heart burn and Acidity:** Heartburn and acidity is common due to hormonal changes and growing uterus presses against your stomach, which can relax your esophageal valve. Avoid overeating, take frequent small meals, sleep in semi reclining position with two pillows. Avoid sleeping immediate after food. You can take antacids to relieves your symptoms.

- **Itching**: Blood supply to your skin increases during pregnancy so there is itching. In advanced pregnancy, abdominal skin stretches and become dry and causes itching. You can apply moisturizer twice daily, wear loose cotton clothes. If itching aggravates then meet your doctor and get yourself checked because it can be symptom of liver disease.
- **Leg cramps:** It occurs due to calcium deficiency more in the night usually in the calf muscles. Elevate your legs while sleeping, ankle movements, exercise and calcium supplements and Vitamin B1 supplement can help. Hot fomentation and massage can also help.
- **Giddiness / syncopal attack:** Standing for long hours or standing abruptly can cause giddiness because less blood gets pooled up in your lower parts of the body and less blood return to your heart resulting in reduced blood flow to brain. So, avoid standing abruptly and standing for long hours.
- **Discharge from nipples:** Colostrum can leak at the end of second and third trimester because your body is preparing for labour. You don't need to worry but if there is decreased fetal movements associated with leaking milk, then consult your doctor. Wear tight breast support.
- **Frequent urination:** In early pregnancy growing uterus presses against your bladder causing you urinate frequently. In later

pregnancy, baby's head presses the bladder and you need to pee frequently. Sometimes you won't be able to empty your bladder fully due to pressure on the bladder so you need to lean forward while urinating in advanced pregnancy.
- **Urinary incontinence:** Sudden leak of urine can occur in later stage of pregnancy while sneezing, coughing, laughing because baby's head is down pressuring the bladder and pelvic muscle also becomes relax.
- **Vaginal discharge:** Vaginal discharge is also common in pregnancy. Clear white discharge without foul smell and itching is normal. But, if you are having greenish, greyish, yellow or curdy discharge associated with foul smell and itching then mostly it is vaginal infection. Maintain hygiene and wear loose cotton underwear and consult your doctor.
- **Swollen legs and ankle:** Venous return to the heart reduces due to growing uterus means, growing uterus presses your veins that return blood from lower limbs to your heart and accumulate in lower part of the body. So, there is swelling in legs and ankle. You can keep your leg elevated by putting over pillow while sleeping. Try to sleep on left side, avoid standing for long hours, do ankle movements.
- **Varicose veins:** Veins in legs and vulva gets swollen because growing uterus presses the

veins that return blood from your legs to the heart. This result in pooling of blood in your veins of legs that swells up and visible. You can apply crepe bandage or compression stockings, elevate your legs while sleeping, avoid standing for long hours, can do ankle movements.

- **Piles / hemorrhoids:** In pregnancy, because of "progesterone hormones" veins in your anus become relax and swollen so they bleed when you have hard stools along with pain. It is annoying but it subsides within a week after birth of your baby. Have lots of fiber rich fruits and vegetables. Do not stand for long hours. You can take sitz bath (sitting in a warm water). Apply lignocaine gel or ice packs.
- **Round ligament pain:** Uterus is supported by round ligament in front on both sides. During pregnancy as your baby grows it get stretched and this causes sharp pain in one side or both sides of pelvic area, more on left side because uterus is shifted more towards right side in pregnancy. Pain is more in the night time because in sleep you change position faster. So, try to turn slowly. You can apply hot bag also. Yoga can also help.

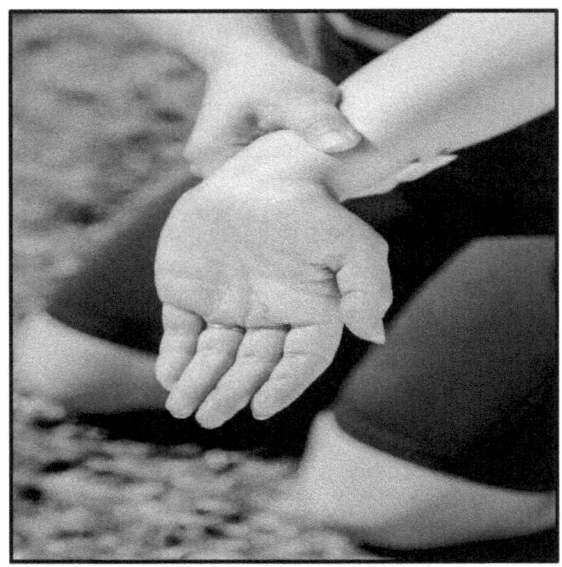

- **Carpel tunnel syndrome:** Due to retention of excess fluid due to hormonal changes in pregnancy there is compression of median nerve leads to pain and numbness in index, middle and thumb. You can apply splint during sleeping, physiotherapy, yoga can also help. It resolves after delivery.

Common problems and its remedies

Sr. No	Problems	Remedies
1.	Cold	Antihistamines, steam inhalation
2.	Nose block	Saline nasal spray, hot shower, steam inhalation
3.	Cough	Gargle with salt water, steam inhalation, honey and lemon in hot water
4.	Fever	Paracetamol
5.	Headache	Paracetamol, consult your doctor because it can be because of high BP.
6.	Leg cramps	Diclofenac gel, leg elevation
7.	Stretch marks	Moisturizer (cocoa butter is the best), olive oil, coconut oil or almond oil
8.	Itching over body	Caladryl lotion or lactocalamine lotion
9.	Itching over genital area	Candid cream, metrogyl cream
10.	White discharge	Clotrimazole vaginal pessary, Betadine vaginal pessary
11.	Piles	Ice pack, lignocaine gel
12.	Carpel tunnel syndrome	Splint, Paracetamol, ice fomentation, physiotherapy
13.	Constipation	Fiber rich diet, isabgol, ghee
14.	Diarrhea	ORS, Probiotics
15.	Indigestion	Antacid, Eno-powder
16.	Toothache	Paracetamol

"You never understand life until it grows inside of you."

— Sandra Chami Kassis

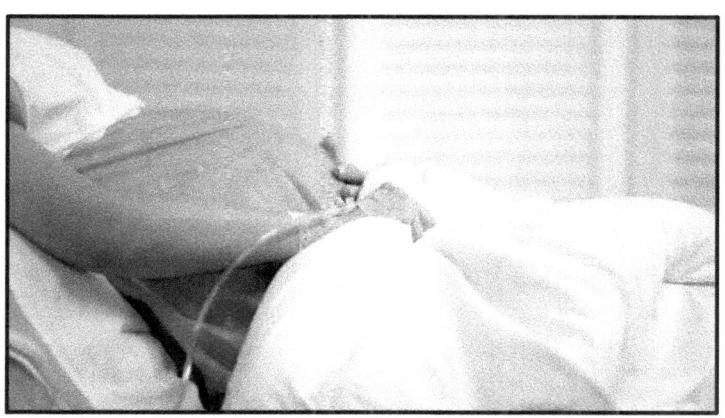

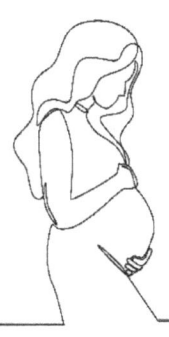

COMMON MEDICAL PROBLEM DURING PREGNANCY

Pregnancy is a physiological state in women's life. Majority of the pregnancy continues till full term without any complications. Sometimes during this physiological process, you may develop some medical problem, which can affect both you and your baby. Most common medical problems are anemia (bloodlessness), hypertension (increase blood pressure) and diabetes (increase blood sugar). One common medical problem which goes unnoticed is urinary tract infection. Now-a-days these medical problems are increasing due to reasons like sedentary pre-pregnancy lifestyle leading to obesity, late age of marriage, use of drugs for conception etc. So you must be aware of these conditions.

- **Anemia**
    - It is the most common medical complication associated with pregnancy.
    - Majority of the women embark into pregnancy with below normal levels of hemoglobin.

- Even if you are non-anemic, you can develop anemia due to normal physiological changes that take place. This usually gets worsen if you don't take proper antenatal care.
- Your Dietary requirement increases to match your physiological change and to maintain your baby's growth.
- Sometimes your diet intake reduces due to vomiting and altered food habits during pregnancy.
- You feel generalized weakness, tiredness, easy fatigability, recurrent infection of urine when you develop anemia.
- If you ignore it can lead to generalized swelling of your body because of less protein and difficulty in breathing because your heart is not functioning properly.

You can prevent this by

- Having your hemoglobin level above 12gm% before you become pregnant.
- Taking an adequate balanced diet during pregnancy.
- Taking supplementary iron and folic acid as advised by your doctor.
- Undergoing appropriate treatment if there is excessive vomiting.
- Undergoing regular antenatal check-up.

- Maintaining personal hygiene to avoid infection e.g., urinary tract infection and worm infestation.

- **Hypertension**
  - You may develop increased blood pressure (hypertension) alone as the pregnancy advances.
  - Sometimes, the condition deteriorates further leading to very high blood pressure and convulsion or fits.
  - If not taken care of it can cause death of either mother or baby or both.
  - Many times, your doctor may not be able to tell you the exact reason for this increase of blood pressure.
  - You are at increased risk of developing this condition if your age is above 35 years, you have conceived with artificial reproductive technique you are overweight you have a family history of high BP i.e., either of parent and you have anemia, diabetes or any other autoimmune diseases.
  - You may gain abnormal weight visible as non-reducible swelling of legs extending towards upper thigh at the begging of this diseases. Sometimes along with this you may experience headache, black flickering in front of your eyes, upper abdominal pain specifically on right side

and reduced urine quantity indicating severity of the condition. You must consult your doctor without delay.

You can prevent it by

- o Undergoing regular antenatal check-up.
- o Avoiding preventable risk factors like anemia and increased weight.
- o Taking adequate calcium supplementation in the presence of risk factors.

- **Diabetes**
  - o The hormonal changes that take place during pregnancy make the you susceptible for developing diabetes.
  - o It can appear at any time during pregnancy.
  - o Majority of the time you may not have any complaints. However, it is detected during the process of routine investigations.
  - o You may notice discharge from vagina with itching and repeated urine infection.
  - o You cannot prevent it. But can detect it and keep it under control by undergoing regular antenatal check-up.
  - o If it is detected you must follow your doctor's advice which will avoid further adverse effect on you and the baby.

- **Urinary Tract Infection**
  - This is the most common infection that occurs during pregnancy.
  - Most of the time you may not have any complaints.
  - Frequency and urgency of urination with lower abdominal pain are the common complaint with this condition.
  - It is usually associated with risk factors like anemia and diabetes.

  This can be prevented by
  - Undergoing regular antenatal check up with repeat urine examination.
  - Maintaining personal hygiene
  - Avoiding preventable risk factors like anemia and diabetes during pregnancy
  - Early detection and treatment will improve the pregnancy outcome.

- **Conclusion**
  - All the above mentioned medical conditions are associated with maternal and fetal complications.
  - If you develop increased blood pressure and diabetes during pregnancy, you are likely to develop the same in future pregnancy and later life also.

- Your baby is also at risk of developing high blood pressure and diabetes when they become adults.
- Although these medical problems are described separately, they may predispose to each other. For example, women with anemia are susceptible to increased blood pressure and urinary tract infection. Similarly, women with diabetes are prone for developing increased blood pressure and urinary tract infection.
- The adverse effects of these medical conditions on pregnancy can be avoided or at least reduced by regular antenatal check-up, taking regular balanced diet and necessary required supplementation

"Pregnancy is the only time when you can do nothing at all and still be productive."

— Evan Esar

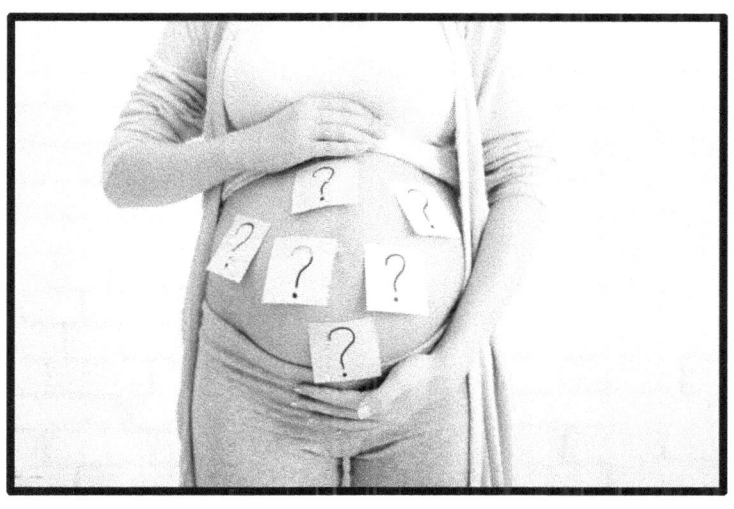

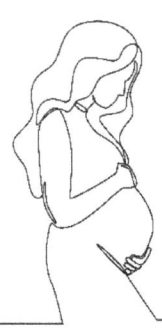

COMMONLY ASKED QUESTION IN PREGNANCY

1. **Will my baby be boy or girl?**

   Everybody wants to know the gender of the baby but in India it's illegal to know the gender of the baby. There are many myths regarding sex prediction like sex positions can predict gender, craving for salty food means boy and craving for sweets means girl child. Well, these are all myths.

   Let's understand science behind this:

   Each cell of human body contains 46 chromosomes except male sperm and female eggs. They contain 23 chromosomes each. Chromosomes are tiny thread like structure which contains approx. 2,000 genes. Genes determines hair and eyes color, height etc. When fertilization occurs, 23 chromosomes of male sperm and 23 chromosomes of female egg become 46. Female has XX chromosomes whereas male has XY chromosomes. If egg is fertilized by sperm containing X chromosomes, then XX (girl) is born whereas when it is fertilized by sperm containing Y chromosomes the XY (boy) is born.

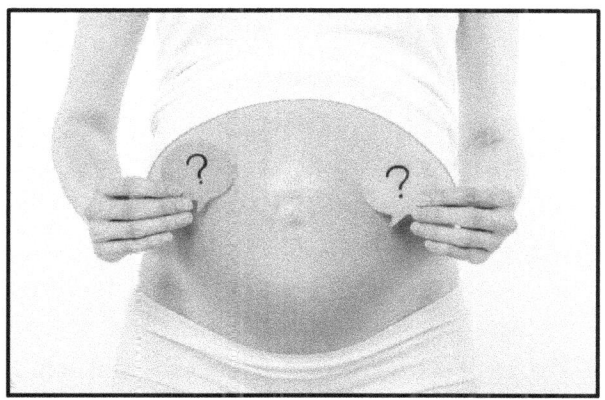

2. How safe is travelling during pregnancy?

Travelling in pregnancy is not harmful for you or for your baby. However, some women prefer not to travel in first trimester because of nausea and vomiting. In third trimester also travelling become tiring and uncomfortable. So women prefer to travel in second trimester. After 37 weeks travelling becomes bit risky because your delivery date is near and you can go into labour any time. Before planning for travelling, consult your doctor for appropriate advice.

- **Timing**
  - Best time to travel is between 14-28 weeks.
  - Avoid travelling after 32 weeks if you have complicated pregnancies with risk factors for

premature labour and twin / triplet pregnancies

- **Duration of traveling:**
  - Long hours of travelling have small chance of getting deep vein thrombosis (DVT), so avoid it. Wear compression stockings which will help in better blood circulation in your legs.
  - While travelling by road don't forget to wear seat belt wherever possible. In case of long hours travel (>2 hours) take some precautions like after certain distance get down off the vehicle and stretch your legs and hands. Walk some distance as well.

- **Mode of transport:**
  - Travelling in train and flight is safer than bike and car because no jerky movements.
  - Air and train travel is not recommended after 36 weeks and if you are travelling then you need to take permission letter from your doctor.
  - Avoid traveling in overcrowded public transport. You may get hurt on your distended abdomen.
  - If you are suffering from cardiac disease, severe anemia respiratory disease, low lying placenta (placenta previa), recurrent bleeding in pregnancy restricts your unwarranted social travel. In case of emergency use ambulance for travel to nearest health facility.

Whenever you are travelling a long distance, don't forget to carry your antenatal reports.

3. What is the probability of delivering on due date?

- Only 4% female deliver on their expected delivery date. 80% deliver two weeks before or 1 week after their due date.

4. What should I do if I am intolerant to iron tablets?

Iron tablets have some gastric side effects like nausea, vomiting etc. If you are not able to tolerate your iron tablets then follow these steps.

- You can avoid taking tablets in empty stomach and take with food or at night.
- You can ask your doctor to give liquid preparation in which it is easy to adjust the dose.
- You can ask your doctor to change the iron tablet preparation which can be taken in between food.
- Ensure intake of iron rich vegetables and fruits like wood apple, banana and dry fruits.

Hope these tips would be helpful to you all my dear readers.

NOTE:

- Iron is better absorbed in your body if taken in an empty stomach.
- Have Vitamin C rich fruits like lemon and oranges.
- Avoid taking your calcium tablets along with iron tablets example if you are taking iron tablet in morning and evening then take calcium tablet in afternoon.
- Avoid taking tea, coffee, milk and bread with iron tablet it reduces its availability.

5. **How to take care of skin care during pregnancy?**

- Blood supply to the skin increases and due to hormonal change your skin looks shinier and plumper.
- Apply moisturizer twice a day which reduce stretch marks and itching due increase blood supply to skin.
- Acnes flare up due to hormonal changes, increased sensitivity and increased oil excretion and dry skin.
- Avoid retinol and salicylic acid for treatment of acne. These drugs can cause congenital malformation.
- There could be hyperpigmentation known as melasma near forehead, cheeks, upper lips and other parts of body even on the folds of body like neck and armpits due to increased

sensitivity to the sun and hormonal fluctuations. This returns to its normal appearance after pregnancy.
o Apply lots of sunscreen to avoid pigmentation and moisturizer for stretch marks. Cocoa butter is best and safe for stretch marks in pregnancy.
o Don't skip your skin routine if you are doing.
o Add Vitamin C serum to your skin care routine. Its antioxidant property, help in skin repair and healing keep your skin glowing and healthy.
o Drink lots of water and have lots of fruits which will keep your skin hydrated and glowing.

6. Why and how to take Dental care in pregnancy?

o Oral health is very important and it should be maintained during pregnancy as well.
o Physiological changes in pregnancy may cause problems like gingivitis, dental caries, tooth mobility. But good oral health keeps your gums and teeth healthy.
o Dental problems like periodontitis are associated with cardiovascular diseases, respiratory diseases, diabetes, low birth weight babies and pre-term labour.
o Consult your dentist if you have not consulted him for last 6 months if you have any dental problems.

- Cleaning, taking x-ray (with shielding of abdomen and thyroid), local anesthesia is safe in pregnancy.
- Problems which require immediate treatment like tooth extraction, root canal, restoration/filling either with silver or composite of untreated caries can be managed at any stage of pregnancy.
- Make a hobbit of brushing your teeth twice a day with fluoridated toothpaste, flossing once a day, dental visit twice a year and limiting sugary food items.

7. What should I do If I feel my baby's movement is reduced?

If you notice your baby's movement is reduced then you must try following things of your own.

- **You can do following things**
  - Have something like juice and walk for sometimes.
  - Stimulate your baby by touching your bump.
  - Shine flashlight on your abdomen

If there is no activity after doing above measures then call your doctor or visit your doctor as soon as possible.

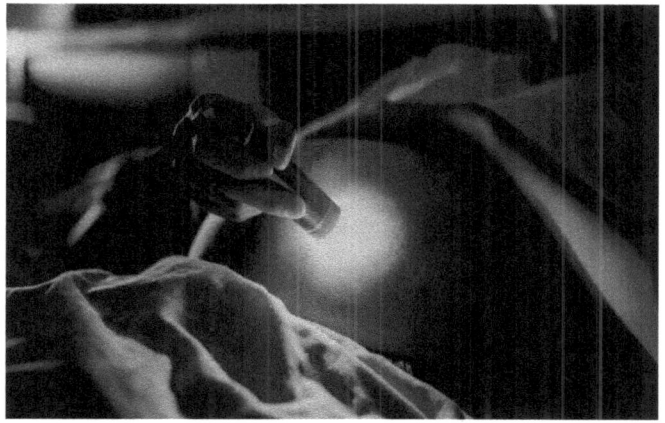

Here are few causes known for feeling of reduced fetal movement.

- If your placenta is anterior then you may perceive less fetal movements. No need to get tensed.
- Your baby may be sleeping. You can caress your bump. Each cycle lasts for 20-40minutes.
- When there low liquor which makes difficult for baby to move.
- Obesity with thick abdominal wall makes difficult for you to perceive fetal movements.
- Low weight/ fetal growth restriction can cause decrease fetal movement.

8. How to count fetal movements?

There are two methods of counting fetal movements. Those are as follows:
- Start counting at a fixed time like example 8am in the morning and as soon as you perceive 10

movements then you can stop. If you perceive 10 movements in 2 to 3 hours then you can stop counting. But if, you don't perceive fetal movements in 2 to 3 hours then you can count for 12 hours. This method is bit difficult.

- You can count fetal movement for 1 hour after each meal i.e., morning, afternoon and night.
- There should be 3 movements in each 1 hour, so there should be total 9 movements. This method is simple.

9. What happens if there is bleeding during pregnancy?

Bleeding is very common in early pregnancy. 15-25% women suffer from vaginal bleeding in early gestation. Bleeding or spotting don't always mean there is a problem but if there is heavy bleeding associated with abdominal pain then there can be chance of miscarriage or other complications.

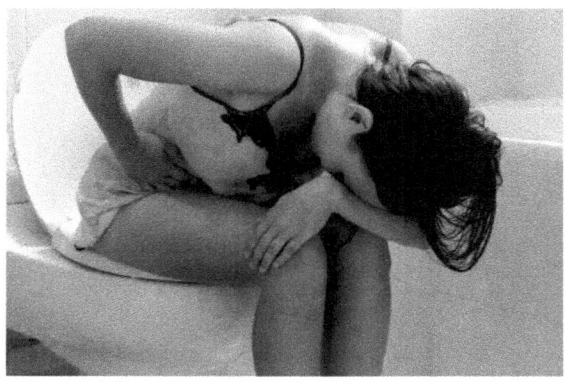

Bleeding/spotting in early pregnancy

- Sometimes it is normal to have spotting/bleeding in early pregnancy which are not associated with abdominal pain or cramp. The reasons are as follows:
- Implantation bleeding- when your embryo attaches to the uterine wall then mild spotting or bleeding can happen and that's absolutely normal. Many patients come to me in first trimester with spotting. I always examine and counsel them.
- Decidual bleeding- This happens due to hormonal imbalance which leads to partial shedding of uterine lining. Its normal. You should not get scared of it.
- Sometimes due to infection and sex during first trimester can cause spotting or bleeding.
- When bleeding is heavy and associated with abdominal pain/cramps, giddiness and weakness, consult or visit your doctor. Keep track of how heavy or light you are bleeding, how many pads you are using, what is the color of your bleeding like dark red or bright red etc., because your doctor will ask all these questions.

Bleeding in advance pregnancy

- Bleeding in later pregnancy can occur after internal examination by your doctor which is normal.

- Bleeding can occur due to infection and sex or labour.
- Some serious problems like pre-term labour (early labour before 37weeks), placenta previa (placenta is low lying) and abruptio placentae (separation of placenta before delivery) can lead to heavy bleeding and danger to the baby as well. In these cases, you need to visit your doctor immediately without delay.

10. If my blood is Rh negative, do I have any problem during pregnancy?

- If you and your husband's blood is Rh-ve type, then you need not worry.
- However, if your blood is Rh -ve and your husband's blood is Rh + then there is 50% chance that your bay will have Rh + fetus. There are possibilities of your baby's blood may enter into your blood circulation. If this happens then your body will make antibodies against that. Those antibodies will cross placenta and enter into your baby's circulation and destroy fetus's red blood cells. This may affect your 1st baby, but it can affect your subsequent baby.
- So, you need to undergo a special blood test known as Indirect coombs test (ICT) at first visit at early pregnancy which is repeated at 24 and 28 weeks.

- If the test is negative, it is good news for you and you should take Anti-D injection between 28-32 weeks to prevent the formation of natural antibodies against fetal blood cell. After delivery also you should take Anti-D injection within 72 hours of delivery if your baby's blood group positive.
- If you couldn't take then you can take within 13 days of delivery.
- If it is positive then, it indicates that you have developed antibodies against your fetus's red blood cells. You need to be followed up in a highly specialized neonatal healthcare facility where your baby can be managed after delivery.

11. How to interact with my baby during ongoing pregnancy?

Emotional connection between you and your baby is very important and it can happen even when your baby is not born. Let's talk about various ways of bonding.

- After 16 weeks your baby can hear you. So, sing, read some book or playing songs loudly to your baby increases brain activity and bond.
- Gentle touch or massage your bump and especially in response to your baby's movement is a great way to interact with your baby and increase the bond with it.

- You can go for yoga class but after 18-20 weeks. Simple stretching and basic poses are safe to do.
- You can do breathing exercise which will calm you down and draws in oxygen down to the baby as well and this oxygen will help your baby become more active, and it will help you pay more attention to your body and help you in connecting to your baby.

12. What to do if water bag breaks!

- First be calm, don't panic!
- Check the color, amount and smell of the liquor. Normal liquor is colorless and it has no smell. If the color of liquor is greenish yellow then it will be meconium stained (fixed with baby's first stool), then it required close monitoring and might need caesarean section as soon as possible.
- Put sanitary pad and note the time of the leak so that it will be easy for you to tell your doctor.
- Try to reach the hospital as soon as possible because in case of delay, chances of infection will increase.

13. How to manage work during pregnancy?

- Pregnancy is very challenging and going to work is even more challenging. So, you need to give extra care at your workplace.

- Avoid strenuous activities during pregnancy like lifting heavy weight, climbing stairs multiple times, standing for long hours etc.
- If you are working with radiation, solvents, toxic chemicals and fumes then you should take break from your work.
- Avoid working more than 8 hours or travelling for long hours for work.
- Wear comfortable shoes and dresses so that you can work comfortably for longer hours.
- Manage stress by doing yoga, breathing exercise or meditation.
- Take regular breaks at least for few minutes and stretch your legs and walk if you are sitting for long hours or if you are standing for long hours then sit, give rest to your back and legs.
- You can wear compression stockings if you have leg cramps or swelling.
- Take maternity leave if you have complications like risk of pre-term labour, placenta previa, cervical insufficiency, fetal growth restriction, pre-eclampsia or uncontrolled diabetes mellitus.

14. Can I have sex during pregnancy?

- Each pregnancy is unique, this activity may vary based on your condition. Here is some general advice for you.
- Sex is considered safe and can continue throughout pregnancy, in most uncomplicated pregnancies.
- If the pregnancy is complicated by bleeding, pain abdomen or prior miscarriage better to abstain from intercourse until it's safe to resume.
- You have open communication with partner regarding understanding of concerns, discomfort, or changes in sexual desire during pregnancy.
- Adequate foreplay and use of water-based lubricants if needed can enhance comfort during intercourse. Pregnancy hormones can affect vaginal lubrication.
- It is safe for a pregnant woman to experience orgasm during intercourse. Contractions which occur during orgasm are usually harmless but may be concerning in specific high-risk situations.
- With the advancement of pregnancy, the size and shape of your belly change, which may affect sexual positions. You need to adopt comfortable positions to avoid putting pressure on the abdomen.

o Gentle and cautious movements are recommended during intercourse to avoid trauma or injury to the abdomen.

15. How to deliver a baby in remote area where hospital facilities are not available or in case of emergency?

Delivering in remote area without facilities can be challenging and safety of mother and baby is more important.

o Stay calm, don't panic!
o Find clean and hygienic place for delivery.
o Get the help of trained birth attendant.
o If possible, call your doctor and take instruction over phone.

"A new baby is like the beginning of all things — wonder, hope, and dream of possibilities."

— Eda J. Le Shan

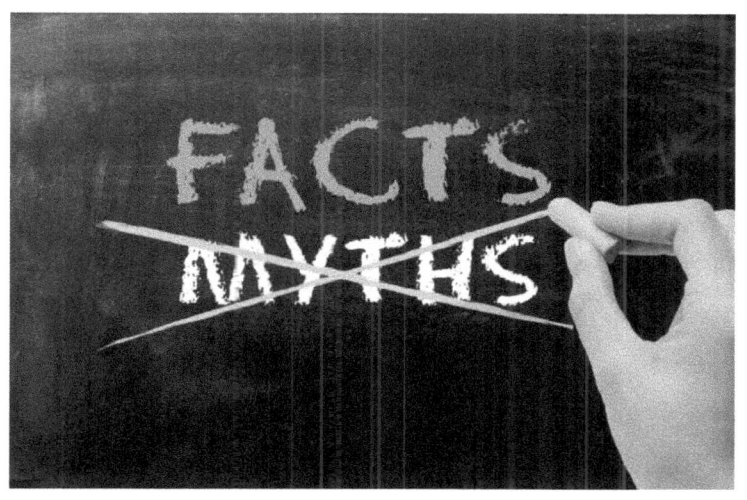

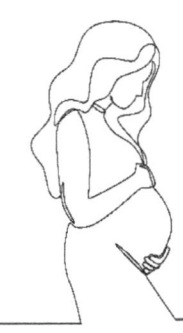

MYTHS AND FACTS RELATED TO PREGNANCY

Pregnancy can be a wonderful and exciting journey, but it's important to separate myths from facts. You can have a **safe and healthy pregnancy** by following accurate information based on scientific research.

Myth 1: Exercise during pregnancy can harm your baby.

- **Fact**: Exercise can be beneficial during pregnancy, as it helps to reduce stress, maintain a healthy weight, and prepare the body for childbirth. You should avoid any exercises that give jolt to your body like racket sports and jumping and jogging. A planned prenatal exercise program is very important to relieve many discomforts of pregnancy and also aids in having a smooth delivery. However, you should consult your healthcare provider before starting or continuing any exercise regimen.

Myth 2: You have to fulfil all your food cravings.

- **Fact**: All expectant mothers develop likes and dislikes towards certain foods. Craving for a particular food is known as "Pica". One should indulge with moderation, as desire for wrong foods may not benefit either the mother or the baby. On the contrary, she may gain a lot of unadvisable weight, which will come in her way of getting back into shape later on.

Myth 3: During the 2nd pregnancy, you do not require any preparation, nor you need exercise.

- **Fact**: Each pregnancy is different and no two labors are alike. Hence, preparation is essential even in your 2nd pregnancy. You need to pay more attention to exercise well so that your muscles do not become slack. Abdominal strengthening will enable you to get the right support for carrying your baby.

Myth 4: You must eat for two people.

- **Fact**: While you need extra nutrients, you only need about 300 extra calories per day. Eating too much can lead to excessive weight gain, which can increase the risk of complications during pregnancy and childbirth.

Myth 5: You should not consume black or dark coloured foods, otherwise your baby's skin colour will be dark.

- **Fact**: Colour of the baby is already determined by the inherited genes and not by the food ingested by you. Many nutritive foods are not eaten because of this false notion.

Myth 6: If your baby is born at night time, he/she will be awake at night.

- **Fact**: Birth time has no relation to the sleeping and waking times of the baby.

Myth 7: If your tummy gets hairy, it's a boy.

- **Fact**: Increase in male hormones during pregnancy lead to hair growth on the belly.

Myth 8: During pregnancy, you always develop a perfect facial glow.

- **Fact**: Not always – Hyper pigmentation, greasy hair and fatigue can occur due to hormonal changes.

Myth 9: All mothers-to-be develop stretch marks.

- **Fact**: Chances of developing stretch marks are 50%. This is generally inherited. If your mother didn't, you may not have them.

Myth 10: If your baby is high – it's a girl. If your baby is low – it's a boy.

- **Fact**: Usually, in first pregnancy, due to good muscle tone, the bump is high. In subsequent pregnancies, the abdominal muscle is slack, the bump will be low.

Myth 11: Big Belly – Big Baby. Small Belly – Small baby.

- **Fact**: A woman with good height may not show too much in spite of the baby being big. In a short statured woman, the belly may look bigger but there is no guarantee of the baby being big.

Myth 12: If you experience heartburns, baby will be born with lots of hair.

- **Fact**: Heartburns occur due to the secretion of gastric juices more frequently by the pressure of growing uterus over the esophagus.

Myth 13: You may be asked to keep secret about your pregnancy in the first trimester to safeguard you and your child from the "evil eye" and not allow a miscarriage to happen.

- **Fact**: The first three months of pregnancy are a little risky for miscarriages, but there is nothing like an "evil eye" to cause a miscarriage !

Myth 14: If your complexion sparkles and you look more beautiful, it's a girl – otherwise a boy.

- **Fact**: The glow and the sparkle are the result of increased blood circulation.

Myth 15: Consuming ghee towards the end of pregnancy will facilitate a smooth and quick delivery.

- **Fact**: Ghee is not essential. Sometimes castor oil is suggested to induce labour. Ghee, butter, oil tend to irritate the intestine causing lose motions. As nerve supply to the intestine and uterus is same, uterine contractions get initiated.

Myth 16: Having sex during pregnancy will result in miscarriage.

- **Fact**: Only in complicated or high-risk pregnancies, abstinence from sex is advised. Otherwise, a pregnant woman can have sexual relations as long as she is comfortable. Details has been motioned in the chapter 'Commonly asked questions in pregnancy'.

Myth 17: Having coconut water after the 7th month will make your baby's hair mushy.

- **Fact**: Coconut water can be consumed as long as the mother wishes to have it. It has no effect on baby's hair.

Myth 18: Baby will be born fair skinned if you consumes saffron milk.

- **Fact**: Baby's complexion and colour is already determined by the genes contribute by you and your husband.

Myth 19: Eating papaya will miscarry the baby.

- **Fact**: Papaya is a healthy food. Large quantities eaten in early part of pregnancy may lead to diarrhea and harmful. After the first trimester, a slice or two can be consumed.

Myth 20: You should have Ghee and Badam Sheera once your labour begins.

- **Fact**: These foods are very heavy and tend to induce vomiting. Also, they take a much longer time to digest; hence emergency caesareans have to wait.

Myth 21: Cord around the baby's neck indicates caesarean delivery.

- **Fact**: A baby with loose loop of cord around the neck can be delivered normally, provided its parameters are normal during labour.

Myth 22: Eat ghee to lubricate the birth passage.

- **Fact**: Exercise is more helpful in increasing the flexibility of the pelvic area. Hence, enroll for a good prenatal class to make labour short and easy.

Myth 23: Pain of childbirth is excruciating and totally unbearable.

- **Fact**: The right preparation done in a prenatal class – physical, emotional and mental will help you to cope up through labour and the breathing techniques will enable you to control these so-called unbearable pains.

Myth 24: Baby gets suffocated if you pull in your stomach.

- **Fact**: Blood circulation to the baby is maintained through the umbilical cord. Pulling in of the abdomen does not restrict this blood flow.

Myth 25: If you are happy and think positive, the baby will grow better.

- **Fact**: **Absolutely true**. Mother's moods have a great effect on the baby. During stress, the body chemistry alters. Hence, try and be cheerful and optimistic throughout pregnancy.

Myth 26: Sitting down on the floor will give rise to premature delivery.

- **Fact**: Squatting for a long time in the early part of pregnancy is not advisable. Sitting on the floor is absolutely harmless and tailor sitting is especially recommended to increase the flexibility and reduce low back pains.

Myth 27: Morning sickness occurs only in the morning.

- **Fact:** Morning sickness can occur at any time of the day or night, and it affects many pregnant women. It is caused by hormonal changes in the body and can be managed with dietary changes, rest, and sometimes medication.

Myth 28: You should avoid all seafood.

- **Fact:** Some types of seafood are high in mercury, which can be harmful to a developing fetus. However, many types of seafood are safe to eat in moderation, and they provide important nutrients such as omega-3 fatty acids.

Myth 29: You should not travel.

- **Fact:** Travel is generally safe during pregnancy, but you should take precautions such as wearing seat belts, staying hydrated, and taking breaks to move around. You should also check with their healthcare provider before traveling, especially if you have any underlying medical conditions. Details has been motioned in the chapter 'Commonly asked questions in pregnancy'.

Myth 30: You should avoid all medications.

- **Fact:** Some medications are safe to take during pregnancy, while others can be harmful. Pregnant women should always check with their healthcare provider before taking any medications, including over-the-counter drugs and herbal supplements.

Myth 31: You should avoid all forms of alcohol

- **Fact:** There is no safe level of alcohol consumption during pregnancy, and even small amounts can increase the risk of fetal alcohol spectrum disorders. You should avoid all forms of alcohol, including beer, wine, and liquor.

Myth 32: You should not get vaccinations.

- **Fact:** Some vaccinations are recommended for pregnant women, such as the flu vaccine and the Tdap vaccine, which protects against tetanus, diphtheria, and pertussis. Vaccines can help to protect both the mother and the developing fetus from serious illnesses. However, live attenuated vaccines are contraindicated during pregnancy.

Myth 33: You should avoid all caffeine.

- **Fact:** Moderate caffeine intake, which is defined as less than 200 milligrams per day, is generally safe during pregnancy. However, excessive caffeine intake can increase the risk of miscarriage and low birth weight.

Myth 34: All women experience the same symptoms during pregnancy.

- **Fact:** Every pregnancy is different, and women can experience a wide range of symptoms during pregnancy. Some women may have no symptoms at all, while others may experience nausea, fatigue, mood swings, and other common pregnancy symptoms.

Myth 35: During pregnancy you can't sleep on your sides.

- **Fact**: You can sleep however you want but it is better to sleep on left side so that blood circulation to your baby is good.

Myth 36: Washing of your navel during pregnancy harm the baby.

- **Fact:** Washing naval during pregnancy is essential to maintain hygiene.

Myth 37: People say caesarean section is easier than normal delivery but this is totally wrong.

- Fact: it is a major surgery which requires longer period for recovery.

Remember to consult with your doctor before making any changes to your diet or exercise routine

Source:

1. https://ninemonthspregnancy.com/common-myths-of-pregnancy/
2. https://neolacta.com/blogs/pregnancy-myths-facts/

"Motherhood is the biggest gamble in the world. It is the glorious life force. It's huge and scary — it's an act of infinite optimism."

– Gilda Radner

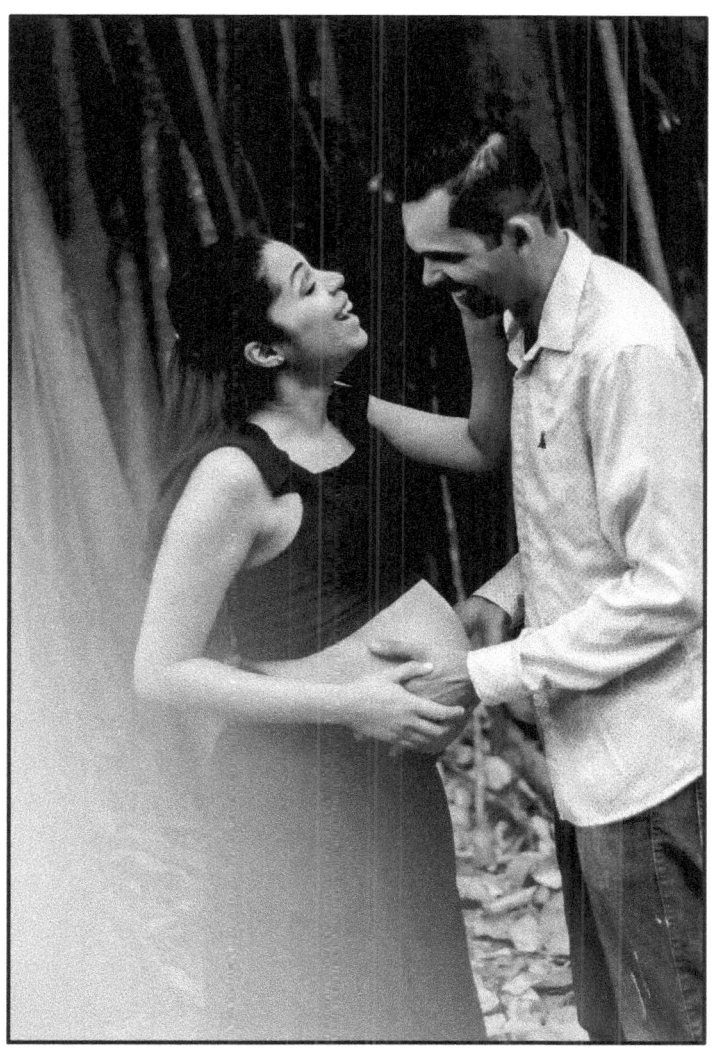

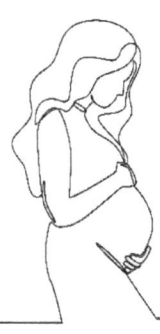

ROLE OF HUSBAND IN PREGNANCY CARE

Pregnancy is a journey that involves physical, emotional, and psychological changes. Husband play a crucial role in your pregnancy care and it is essential also. This can significantly impact you and your baby's well-being. Having a supportive partner can make a significant difference in the overall experience. Here are some key aspects of your husband's role in your pregnancy care:

- **Emotional support:** Pregnancy can be an emotionally challenging time for the expectant mother. Hormonal fluctuations, physical changes, and concerns about the baby's health can lead to anxiety and stress. Being emotionally supportive, understanding, and actively listening to your feelings and concerns can be incredibly beneficial to you.
- **Accompanying during medical appointment:** Attending prenatal check-ups and medical appointments with you shows involvement and care. It allows your husband to stay informed about your pregnancy's progress, understand your and

baby's the health. It also allows his active participation in decision-making regarding your pregnancy.

- **Educating and learning together:** Educating oneself about pregnancy, childbirth, and new-born care is crucial for both of you. This shared knowledge helps in making informed decisions, understanding what to expect during the different stages of pregnancy, and preparing for the arrival of the baby.
- **Assisting with household works:** As the pregnancy progresses, you may experience physical discomfort and fatigue. Assisting with household chores, especially tasks that may be challenging for your pregnancy, can be immensely helpful.
- **Healthy lifestyle support:** Supporting a healthy lifestyle is vital during your pregnancy. This includes encouraging a balanced diet, regular exercise (as advised by healthcare providers), and avoiding harmful substances like tobacco, alcohol, and certain medications that can adversely affect your baby's development.
- **Offering physical comfort:** Providing physical comfort, such as offering back rubs or massages, can help alleviate your pregnancy-related aches and pains.
- **Preparing for labour and childbirth**: Attending childbirth education classes together and discussing birthing preferences can help your

husband understand the process of labour and childbirth, as well as contribute to a positive birthing experience.
- **Building a support network:** Engaging in discussions about pregnancy with friends, family, and other expectant couples can help build a support network for both of you.
- **Bonding with the baby:** During pregnancy, your husband can bond with the baby by feeling your baby's movements, talking or singing to the baby, and actively participating in preparations for your baby's arrival.
- **Being there during labour and delivery:** Being present during labour and childbirth, providing encouragement, and offering physical and emotional support during this intense experience can be a tremendous source of comfort for you.

Overall, your husband's active involvement and support throughout the pregnancy journey can contribute to a healthier, happier pregnancy experience for you and your baby. It's essential for both of you to communicate openly, share responsibilities, and face the challenges of pregnancy together as a team.

"A man is not complete until he has seen the baby he has made."

— Sammy Davis Jr.

www.ingramcontent.com/pod-product-compliance
Lightning Source LLC
LaVergne TN
LVHW061550070526
838199LV00077B/6977